The Book of Tomorrow

Inspirational Insights for Rebuilding Civilization

Copyright ©2025

All rights reserved, No part of this book may be reproduced, in any form or by any means, without permission in writing from the author or publisher, except for brief excerpts used in reviews.

TABLE OF CONTENTS

TABLE OF CONTENTS 3

THE MOST IMPORTANT THING 8

HOW THE EARLY PIONEERS BUILT THE SELF- FEEDING FIRE   11

What You'll Need 12
How to Build the Self-Feeding Fire Fast 12
Tips 14

THE SURVIVAL FOOD OF THE U.S. CIVIL WAR - HOW TO MAKE HARDTACK BISCUITS   15

Ingredients 17
Hardware 17

LOST PIONEER RECIPES FROM THE 18TH CENTURY 22

Mud Apples 22
Gorge Pasta 22
Hot Water Cornbread 23
Sweet Potatoes in Cream and Butter 23

HOW NORTH AMERICAN INDIANS AND EARLY PIONEERS MADE PEMMICAN   24

Nutritional Qualities 25
Directions 26
   Ingredients 26
   1. Rendering the Fat 26
   2. Dried Meat Preparation 30
How Much Do I Need? 34

HOW THE SHERIFFS FROM THE FRONTIERS DEFENDED THEIR VILLAGES AND TOWNS .. 35

Crime in the West 36
Equipment 37
Organization 39
The Sheriff 40
Deputy Sheriffs 40
Posses 40
Bringing it up to date 41
Showing the Flag 42
Raising a posse 43

SPYCRAFT 45

MILITARY CORRESPONDENCE DURING THE 1700S TO 1900S 45

Rectal Acorn, Silver Ball, and Quill Letters 45
Invisible Ink 46
Mask Letters 48

WILD WEST GUNS FOR SHTF AND A GUIDE TO ROLLING YOUR OWN AMMO ... 50

- Modern Firearms ... 50
- Handguns ... 51
- Rifles ... 51
- Ammunition ... 52

Reloading Components ... 53
- The Cartridge Case ... 53
- Processing Brass Cartridge Cases ... 54
  - Primer Pocket ... 54
- Bullets and Projectiles ... 55

The Cast Lead Bullet ... 55
Casting Bullets ... 56
- The Bullet Mold ... 56
- The Lead Melting Pot ... 56
- The Ladle ... 57
- The Melting Process ... 57
- The Casting Process ... 57
- Swaging Bullets ... 58
- Machining Bullets ... 59
- The Final Word on Lead Bullets ... 59

Powder ... 59
- Black Powder ... 59
- Smokeless Powder ... 60

Primers ... 60
- Primer Size ... 60

HOW OUR ANCESTORS MADE HERBAL POULTICE TO HEAL THEIR WOUNDS ... 61

What is a Poultice? ... 61

A Few Poultice Recipes ... 63
- Cataplasma Aromaticum ... 63
- Soothing Poultice ... 63
- For Stomach Aches ... 64
- A Mustard Poultice ... 64
- A Native American Recipe to Treat an Abscess ... 64
- A Word of Warning from The Past ... 65

WHAT OUR ANCESTORS WERE FORAGING FOR OR HOW TO WILDCRAFT YOUR TABLE .. 66

- Arrowhead (Sagittaria Latifolia) ... 66
- Asparagus (Asparagus Officinalis) ... 67
- Bulrush (Scirpus acutus, Scirpus validus) ... 68
- Cattails (Typha Latifolia, Typha angustifolia) ... 69
- Chickweed, Common ... 70
- Chicory (Cirhorium Intybus) ... 71
- Cleavers ... 72
- Dandelion (Taraxacum Officionale) ... 73
- Henbit (Lamium Amplexicaule) ... 74
- Lady's Thumb (Polygonum persicaria) ... 75

HOW OUR ANCESTORS NAVIGATED WITHOUT USING A GPS SYSTEM..................................76
- Shadow Tip Method 76
- Watch Method 77
- Using the Stars 77
- Letting the Sun Guide You 78
- Letting the Moon Guide You at Night 79
- Moss and Other Vegetation 79
- Making a Compass 79

HOW OUR FOREFATHERS MADE KNIVES 80
- **Forging a Knife Blank** 81
  - Forging the Blade 81
  - Forging the Tang 81
- **Grinding the Blade** 82
- **Hardening the Blade** 82
- **Making the Handle** 84
- **To Make Your Own Knife** 84

GOOD OLD FASHION COOKING ON AN OPEN FLAM...86
- **Cast Iron Cooking** 86
  - Care and Use 87
- **Roasting Meats** 88
  - On a Spit 88
  - On a String 89
- **Dutch Oven Cooking** 90
  - The Right Temperature 91
  - Companion Tools 91
- **Recipes Past and Future** 92
  - Colcannon 92
  - Meat Pies 92

LEARNING FROM OUR ANCESTORS HOW TO PRESERVE WATER........................96
- How Can I Make Sure That the Water Is Clean? 99
- Where Should I Hide or Store My Stock of Water? 101

HOW AND WHY I PREFER TO MAKE SOAP WITHMODERN INGREDIENTS.........103
- History 103
- Why Modern Ingredients 104
- Understanding The Process 104
- Irreplaceable Ingredients 104
- Machinery and Equipment for Making Soap at Home 105
- Possible Soap Additives 105
- Essential Oils 106
- So, How do You Make Soap? 106
- Methodology 107

TEMPORARILY INSTALLING A WOOD-BURNING STOVE DURING EMERGENCIES............110
- Why a Wood-Burning Stove 110
- Temporarily Installing Your Wood-Burning Stove 111
- Temporarily Installing the Chimney 112
- Heating with Wood 112

MAKING TRADITIONAL AND SURVIVAL BARK BREAD..114
- How to Make Sourdough Starter (The Rising Agent People Used Before 1900)   115
- How to Make Tasty Bread Like in 1869 116
- Making Bark Bread (Famine Bread) 117

HOW TO BUILD A SMOKEHOUSE AND SMOKE FISH...119
- Cold Smoking 119
- Before We Start: Woods for Flavoring Your Fish 119
- Cold Smoking the Fish 119
- First Things First: Curing the Fish 119
- Making a Cold Smoker 121
- Creating the smoker 121
- Hot Smokin'! 124
- Recipes Using Smoked Fish 125

LEARNING FROM OUR ANCESTORS HOW TO TAKE CARE OF OUR HYGIENE WHEN THERE ISN'T ANYTHING TO BUY.. 126
- **Soap Making** 126
  - Basic Recipe for Soap 127
  - Making Lye Water from Wood Ash 127
- **Homemade Toothpaste**.. 128
  - Basic Baking Soda Recipe 128
  - Clay Toothpaste 128
  - To Taste 128

HOW OUR FOREFATHERS MADE SNOW SHOES FOR SURVIVAL.............................129
- **Anatomy of a Snowshoe**... 129
- **Making Survival Snowshoes** 130
- **Using Your Snowshoes** 131

HOW OUR FOREFATHERS BUILT THEIR SAWMILLS, GRAIN MILLS AND STAMPING MILLS 132
- How the Overshot Wheel Works 133
- Making That Force Usable 135
- Gears 135
- Belts 137
- For Reciprocating Saws 137
- Don't Forget Lubrication 138
- Building Your Own Water Wheel 139

The most important thing

I grew up with parents who were already quite advanced in age, and my grandparents were born in the late 1800s. As a result, I was raised in a world that seemed out of step with modern times—an upbringing that was decidedly 'old-school.'

The stories my parents and grandparents shared were from a time so different from today. They talked about making do with what little they had and finding contentment in simplicity. My mother often reminisced about how wealthier families would pass down clothing to less fortunate children, who would be excited to receive these "new" hand-me-downs. My brother and I would return home after school to a warm bowl of soup at my grandparents' house, made from yesterday's leftovers and butcher scraps. It remains the best soup I've ever had. Their lives reflected a different era and a completely different mindset.

Here we are, in the 21st century, worlds apart from our grandparents' way of life. Are we really better off now? Has modern technology made life better than what they had? I doubt it. I see a world where people expect everything to be handed to them, where consumerism has taken over, and where owning the latest gadget is seen as a necessity. Many can't even function without constant access to the Internet.

It's almost paradoxical that we talk about the Internet as something that 'connects the world.' The Internet of Things (IoT) promises an interconnected web of humans and devices, but in reality, we've never been so disconnected from what really matters—our environment, our communities, and even ourselves.

We've lost the ability to take care of our loved ones and ourselves. We depend so much on faceless companies to fulfill our every need that many can't even cook a basic meal anymore, relying on takeout and processed foods instead. This dependency has also affected our health, both mental and physical. What we need now is reconnection—reconnecting with each other and with the natural world. We must rediscover the skills our grandparents had, the skills that saw them through tough times like wars and famines.

The shift in attitudes and expectations between their generation and ours is stark. Our grandparents didn't have the luxury of indulgence that we take for granted today. They lived frugally, knowing that resources were limited.

My grandmother didn't own a wardrobe full of clothes. She would make her own—buying fabric, creating patterns from existing garments, cutting, and sewing them herself. She was an expert knitter and made clothing for the entire family. When something tore or wore out, it was mended, not discarded. This wasn't a trend like today's recycling or upcycling movements; it was simply a way of life.

My grandfather grew vegetables, fished, and bartered for meat. These homegrown foods were essential to my mother's childhood. Meat was a rare treat, not an everyday staple like it is now. Home remedies were also common, as they couldn't afford frequent trips to the doctor. From herbal teas to poultices, they used natural methods to treat various ailments. As modern medicine faces challenges like antibiotic resistance, these old remedies may once again become relevant.

These skills were passed down through generations. My mother learned to sew and knit from an early age and turned it into her livelihood. Folk medicine recipes and knowledge of wild berries were taught to children so they could fend for themselves. We need to return to that spirit of self-sufficiency, to say, "I can take care of myself and my family. I don't need material things for the sake of having them. What I need is health, happiness, and connection."

Our planet is at a tipping point. With over seven billion people on Earth and growing, we are taking more from the planet than it can sustain. The Anthropocene era has begun—a time when human activity is changing the environment in irreversible ways.

The day may come when these old skills, passed down from our grandparents, become crucial again. A major crisis—whether it's an EMP, war, or some other disaster—could force us to relearn the survival skills we've long neglected. Many people, detached from real life and dependent on modern conveniences, won't make it.

We'll have to replace social media with genuine community. Instead of buying things we don't need, we'll embrace the "make do and mend" mentality of our ancestors. We'll rediscover the joys of using our hands, minds, and bodies to truly live in and explore the world, rather than passively consuming it.

Yes, I was raised in an old-fashioned way, but those of us who can grow our own food, heal ourselves, and build our own homes may find that these skills offer invaluable security in a future that looks increasingly uncertain.

HOW THE EARLY PIONEERS BUILT THE SELF- FEEDING FIRE

- By James Walton –

"Some Native people suggest that one shouldtest how cold the hands are by touching the thumb to the little finger of the same hand. As soon as you cannot carry out this exercise you are reaching a dangerous state of incapacity and you should immediately take steps to warm up." – M. Kochanski

Spanning some 300 years from the first contact ofsettlers in Jamestown pioneers have explored their way across this massive continent. The pioneers pushed westward and touched every part of this great land. Farmers, fur traders, miners and surveyors all played a crucial role in expanding the nation.

All that said these men were not staying at the Holiday Innduring their explorations. Pioneers were surviving out in the elements. Whether Summer or Winter these brave menand women forged on against the worst the North American climate could throw at them. On this nasty road self-reliance was everything.

It took a great deal of ingenuity to battle the elements, the wildlife, the germs and the Indians as these pioneers traveled on their way. Things like sewing, weaving, canningand gunsmithing were skills that simply had to be learned when you were surrounded by thousands of miles of hostilewilderness. Of course they paid special attention to the survival basics water, fire and shelter were prioritized above all else.

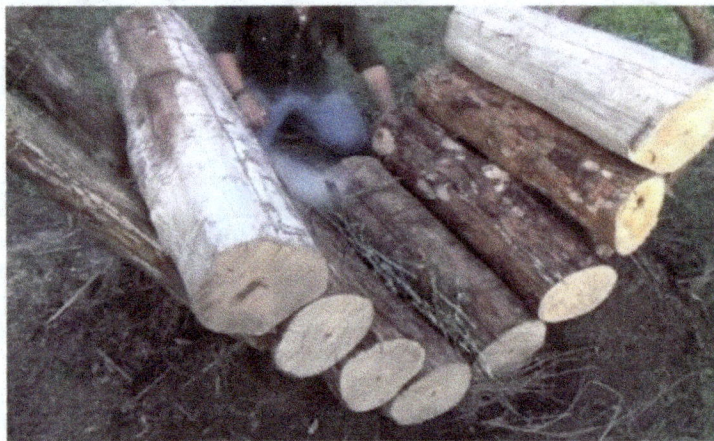

The self-feeding fire was the pioneers answer to getting some sleep at night and not having to constantly tend to a typical campfire. This method of creating a fire utilizes the power of gravity to feed the fire fresh logs. These logs are stacked over one another on two small ramps that roll the logs into one another. The ramps are held up by two large braces and the whole structure is bound together by paracord.

What You'll Need

- 4 small tree trunks or large straight tree branches (about 5 ft. in length)
- 4 branches or smaller trees that will support the larger branches
- 2 branches about 2ft long that will be used in your bracing structure
- 8 large 3ft long sections of tree trunk, preferably hardwood
- 2 small pieces of wood to space your starting logs
- 50 yards of 50/50 chord
- Plenty of dry kindling
- A shovel

The first step in the process is to gather your materials to build the structure itself. Be sure that the materials you gather or cut down are sturdy and strong as this structure will be holding some serious weight. Look for similar sized tree trunks or freshly fallen trees to create the V shape that will be filled with your fuel for the fire.

How to Build the Self-Feeding FireFast

You will start by creating the braces using your four smaller branches and your 2ft branches. They will be lashed together with your paracord.

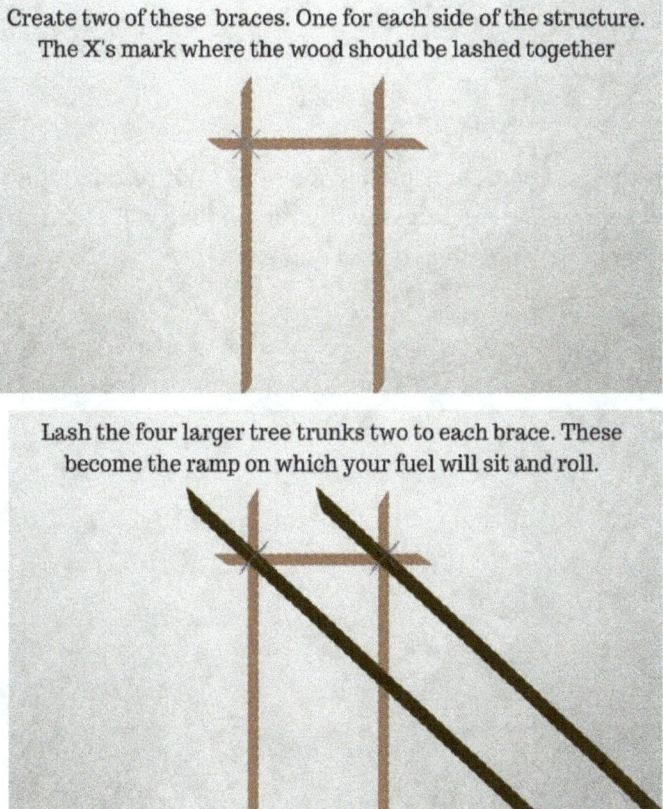

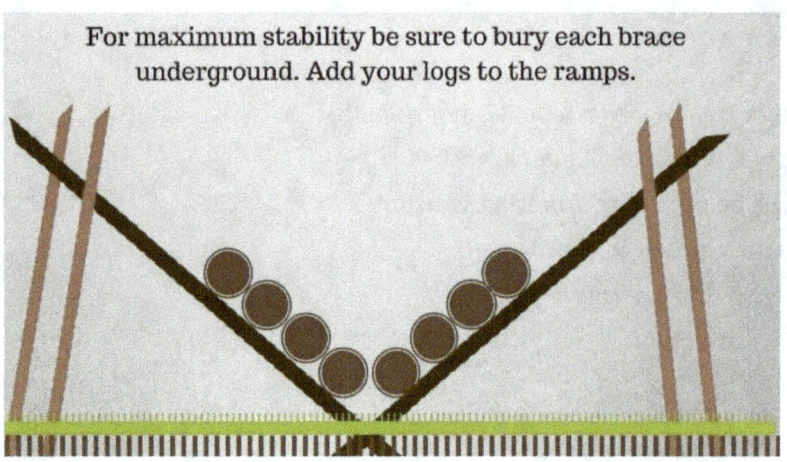

For maximum stability be sure to bury each brace underground. Add your logs to the ramps.

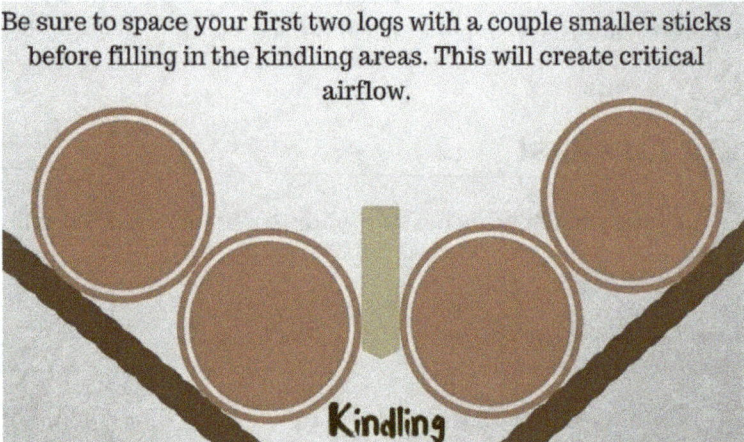

Be sure to space your first two logs with a couple smaller sticks before filling in the kindling areas. This will create critical airflow.

To light the fire place your kindling in the area marked kindling above. Do not remove the spacers that you have put in place. Allow them to burn away as well. Success with your kindling will mean that your first two logs are burning tight against one another. It may not be a roaring flame but there will be an assuring orange glow that will burn for hours.

If your fire smolders out before the main logs start burning all is not lost. The quick fix is to space your logs again with a couple new sticks and fill the areas with new kindling again. We are not pioneers nor are we left to their challenges so if you are really struggling help this thing along with some kind of accelerant.

The self-feeding fire will easily burn for 8+ hours allowing you a great sleep without stoking flames and adding logs. This forgotten skill is but a testament to what the human race is able to derive from adversity. It's not as easy as throwing together a quick campfire but I can promise you when you wake up warm to the sun creeping over the horizon and a fire still burning for breakfast it will all be worth it.

Tips

- Build your base of sturdy materials and don't chince on your paracord
- Be sure to bury all of the legs of your structure that touch the ground.
- The early stages of the fire will be all about oxygen, provide airflow
- Use several sizes of kindling and distribute through the length of the first two log.
- When in doubt use an accelarant!

THE SURVIVAL FOOD OF THE U.S. CIVIL WAR - HOW TO MAKE HARDTACK BISCUITS

- By James Walton -

"An army marches on its stomach"

– *Napoleon Bonaparte*

Though it may have been fire that brought humans out of the darkness and into the light. Just as powerful was the advent of agriculture that allowed us to build communities and stop running and gunning for survival.

Buried in the heap of incredible technologies that catapulted our race to the very moon itself lies an often neglected staple. It was an invention that would have made sea exploration nearly impossible. It was a food that fed soldiers at war for thousands of years. I'm talking about Hardtacks.

Not familiar with name? Well, it goes by many others as well. The fact of the matter is this staple of the seafaring peoples of old and pioneers alike has been called cabin bread, pilot bread, sea biscuit, sea bread, ship's biscuit and as we will discuss now, hardtack.

The journey across the Atlantic was a harsh one that required a food source that could last the long journey. The hardtack offered a carbohydrate energy source that was simply void of moisture. This dried mixture of flour and water was often baked as many as 4 times to assure it could be stored for years if needed without spoiling.

That said the hardtacks were not bullet proof. There are stories of sailors opening barrels of hardtack only to find armies of beetles waiting inside and their food storage for the voyage squandered. But these stories were very uncommon. At Wentworth Museum (Pensacola, Florida) you can find a Hardtack still edible from the U.S. Civil War -1862.

In Alaska, people still eat hardtacks and actually enjoy them! Though the hardtack eaten in Alaska today is not coming from the recipe we will discuss here… it's still a very simple leavened version with the addition of some fat as well.

Survival kits are required cargo on flights by light aircraft in Alaska and it seems these hardtacks are a favorite addition to these kits, so much so that they are available everywhere these flights land or takeoff.

During the civil war the South was strangled by a naval blockade that kept fresh wheat out of the hands of the Confederacy. In fact, in the early days of the war the army was eating hardtacks from the Mexican American war, which ended in 1848. This astounding fact should drive home the effectiveness of this food.

It was not uncommon for a soldier's full meal to consist of one hardtack for breakfast, one hardtack for lunch and one for dinner. Now consider the grueling hikes and hand to hand combat that ensued. These warriors of our past fought it out with little more than coffee and flour in their stomachs.

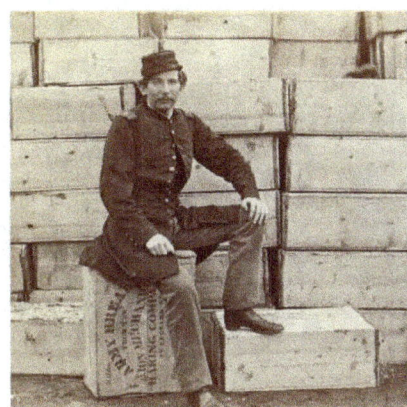

Though the Union army had more resources their soldiers, too, had to depend on hardtacks as well. Of course they were not eating biscuits from previous wars yet these were still rock hard.

To temper its hard nature, they would often dip it into coffee, whiskey or tea. This acted as a softener. Some of the men were smashing them with rifle butts and mixing in river water to make a mush. If a frying pan was available, the mush could be cooked into a lumpy pancake. If not, it was dropped directly on campfire coals.

For dessert, hardtack was sometimes crumbled with brown sugar and hot water. If whiskey was available, that was added. The resulting dish was called a pudding.[3]

The best place to find real honest hardtacks being made is at the popular civil war reenactments. The men and women who participate in the historic battles often enjoy producing some of the foods of that time. These hardtacks produced by the enactors will be the most authentic you can find outside of making them in your own kitchen.

Hardtacks are also gaining popularity among preppers and survivalists. The tough biscuit is prized for exactly the same reasons it was in the past. There is an understanding that if it all goes bad these things will be around. Though they may not be the most delicious option they could feed you and your family in a bad situation. Thus hardtacks are becoming part of an extensive inventory of long term food storage.

The brilliant thing about hard tacks is that they are little more than water, flour and salt. This is why they last an eternity. The desire to add things for flavor and texture is alluring but remember the true purpose of this food is to last forever! The addition of things like fats that can go rancid will shorten the lifespan of this food.

I will provide you with a basic recipe for creating these biscuits. What's more important, however, is that you understand the basic ratio. Many people think cooking is about recipes but really to know a ratio is much more

---
[3] According to historian William Davis

powerful than a recipe because it can be manipulated easily. The ratio for hard tacks is 3:1 flour to water. This canbe 3 cups of flour to 1 cup of water or 3lbs to 1lb or 3 tons to 1 ton. Take this ratio and apply it any way you see fit.

Ingredients

- 3 cups of flour
- 1 cup of water
- 2 teaspoons of salt

Hardware

Cookie sheet or pizza stone ($9 ceramic planter bottom atthe local home and garden store)

- Large mixing bowl
- Rolling pin
- Pizza cutter (not necessary)
- Fork
- Big nail

Preheat the oven to 350 degrees.

Add your flour to the large mixing bowl and stir it around abit with your fork.

Add the salt to your bowl next and make sure that it getswell integrated into the mix.

One of the best pieces of advice I can give you when making dough by hand (and if you're making hard tacksleave the food processor in the cupboard) is to make a

well. Once all of your dry ingredients are incorporated create a hole in the center of the flour. Use your fork topush the flour up and around the edges of the bowl.

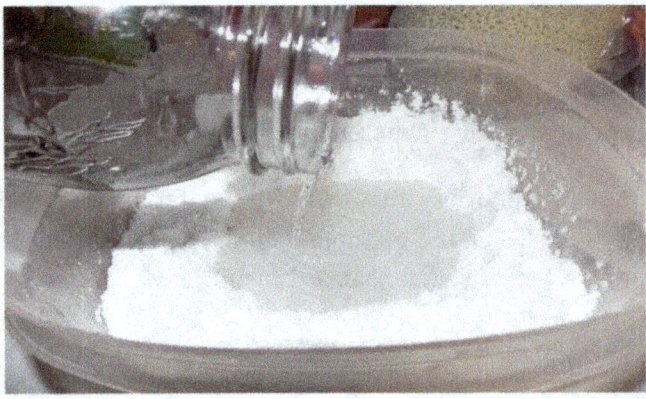

Pour your water into the well and slowly begin to incorporate the flour into the water. With your fork slowly knock the sides into the well allowing the water to begin to thicken. This technique with the well allows you to control how much flour you add into your mixture.

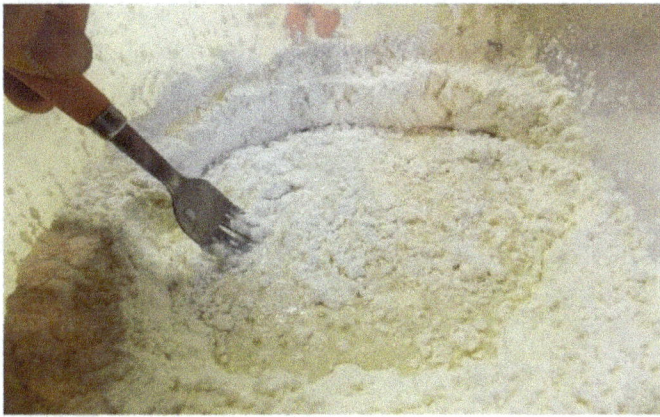

Once the mix gets stodgy and doughy you can turn it out onto a floured table. This mass will still be pretty stick and it will take some additional flour and elbow grease to make it smooth.

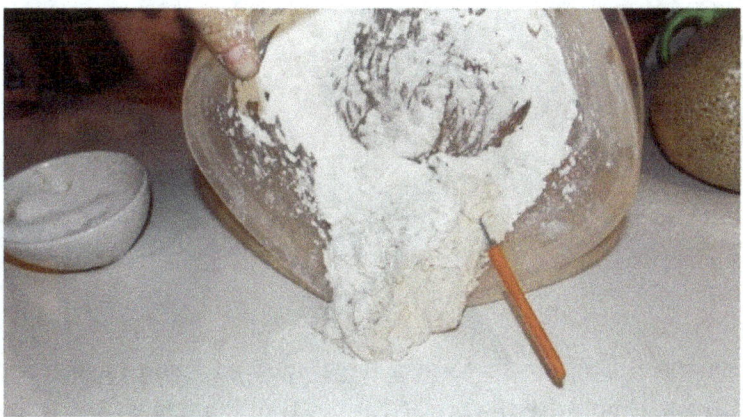

Begin to work the dough by poking at it with your finger tips and folding it over itself. Add flour until it stops sticking to the table and your hands. The dough will get smooth and soft after just a couple minutes.

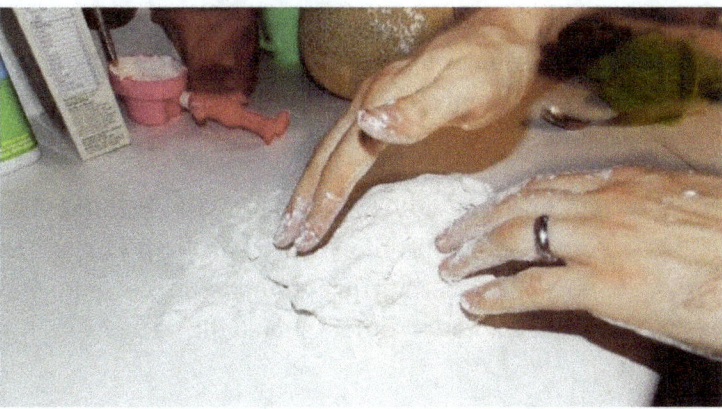

Once your dough has come together you can begin to round it out. You want smooth dough that won't stick to your rolling pin or whatever else you use to shape your hardtack. The picture below shows our dough ready for the next steps.

There are several ways you can manipulate your hardtacks into various shapes. I utilize the rolling pin and the pizza cutter. You could go as crazy as to use a cookie cutter. Just know that although they may be shaped like

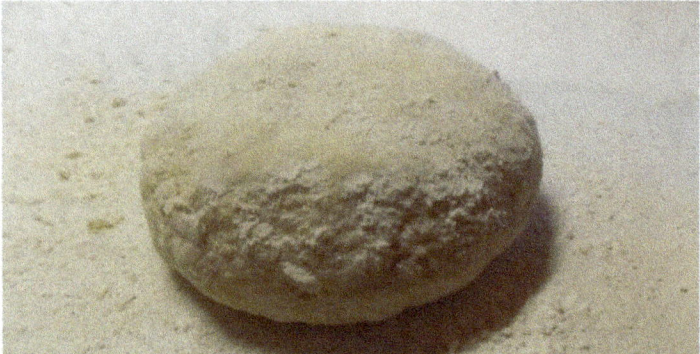

dinosaurs these tough biscuits will not soon become a favorite around the house.

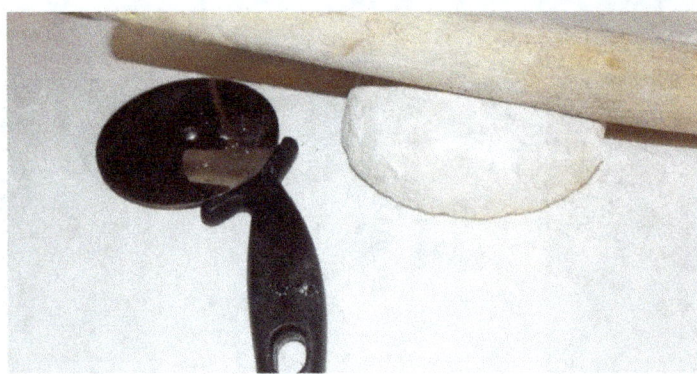

One method for forming hardtacks is to use the rolling pin to form a large square. If you have trouble forming the square from your round ball of dough, simply use the pizza cutter to trim the edges. Assure your hardtacks are at least 1/2 inch thick. Remember these things were actually dinner for the soldiers of the Revolution, Civil War, and maybe even the Roman Legions.

Utilize a common household nail to poke holes into the hard tack. This allows the center of your biscuit to dry out quicker and more thoroughly in the oven. For a nice sized square hardtack poke 16 holes straight through the dough.

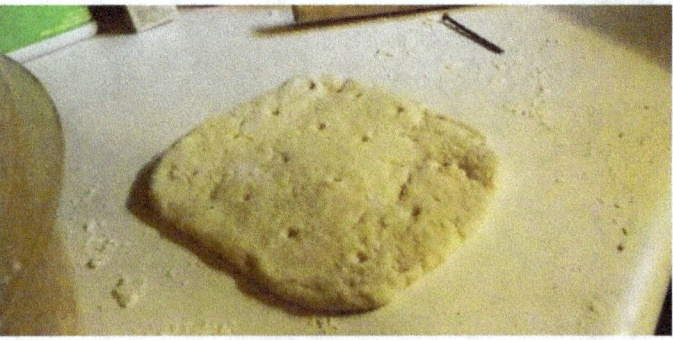

Another method for shaping your hardtacks is to break your dough down into smaller portions. These portions will cook quicker and can be more easily divided amongst others should the need arise.

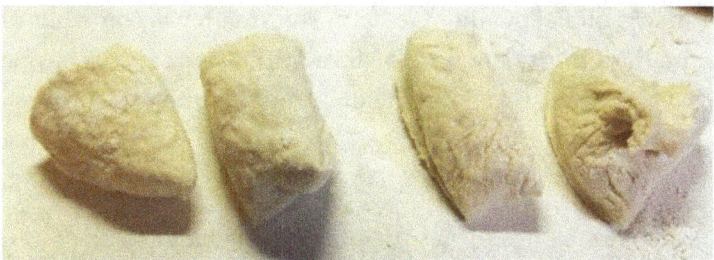

From here shape the portions into smaller circles. These will become your individual portions. Though smaller than the large square method featured above these will also need holes punched in them using the nail.

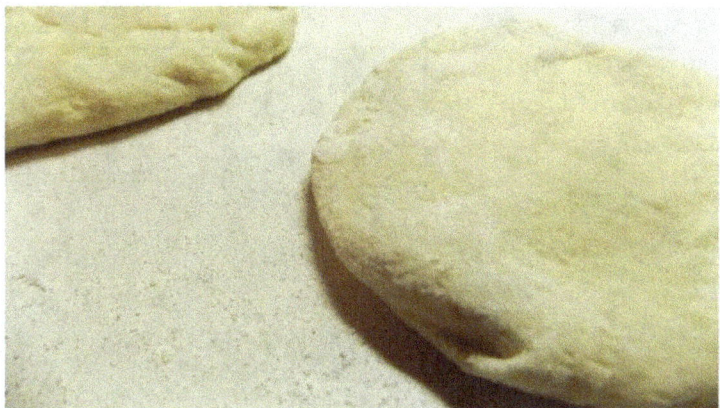

When you think about this ancient recipe and how it must have been prepared all those years ago it's really hard to throw these things on a teflon coated cookie sheet and bake them like chocolate chip cookies. Invest in a clayplanter bottom at your local home and garden store.

These are an incredible tool for baking breads or making stellar pizza out of a home oven. They cost about $9.00 and last a long time. The clay is highly effective because it holdsheat so well.

Lay your hardtacks out and give them enough space to bakeevenly. Place them in the oven for 30 mins.

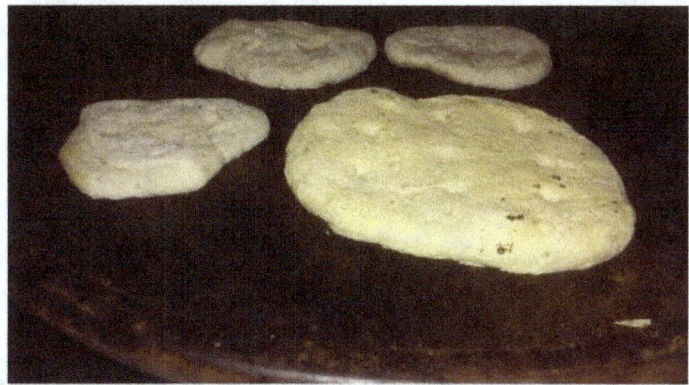

This 30-minute cook time is merely the first of at least two bakes these hard biscuits will go through. This process, although time consuming, will assure that there is no remaining moisture in your hardtacks. Any moisture becomes the complete enemy of this process of shelf stability. Some old recipes call for 3 and even 4 times in theoven. These biscuits must have been closer kin to bricks than food.

Once your first 30 minutes is over pull out the hardtacks and allow them to cool. The steam will come out of them and they will get pretty hard. They will not be hard or dry enough to store at this point. After having cooled them for about 20 minutes place them back in the oven. This time set your timer for one hour.

It will be this bake that thoroughly dries your biscuits and also begins to give them a pleasing bit of color.

Following the last hour of baking turn your oven off. DO NOT REMOVE THE HARDTACKS. Leave your pilot's biscuits in the off turned oven. Let the heat slowly drop in the oven while your biscuits slowly dry even further. This is a great practice for really zapping any remaining moisture left inside.

By this point you have created some decent shelf stable hardtacks. Now unlike most foods you spend time making from scratch I can say you will be delighted to try them. You see they are dry and hard. Those are basically the two features for your palate when it comes to hardtacks.

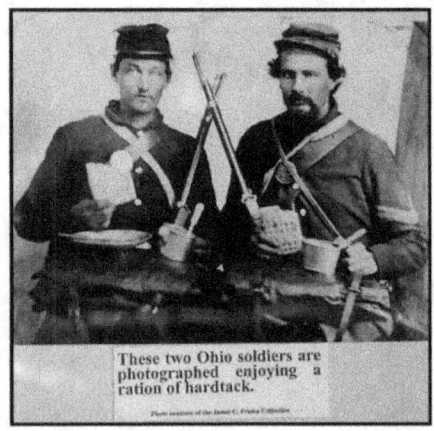

These two Ohio soldiers are photographed enjoying a ration of hardtack.

It won't get much better than that and really it shouldn't. Remember if you decide to flavor them up with butter or herbs this will simply add ingredients that will drastically shorten the shelf life of your hardtacks. Keep it simple and they will last forever.

Also, when you read about just how hard these HARDtacks are you must understand there aren't words that do them justice. If you do decide to taste the fruits of your labor, I advise you to take some precautions. Make sure you are chewing with the best teeth you have. If there is anything loose or filled in there it may very well come out or even shatter.

All jokes aside this is an ancient food that has carried entire nations through tough times. If you follow the recipe above and store your hardtacks properly there is no doubt these biscuits will do the same for you and your family. Of course, if that day ever comes.

LOST PIONEER RECIPES FROM THE 18TH CENTURY

"You don't need a silver fork to eat good food."

-Paul Prudhomme

Whether pushing west into the dangerous and unknown territories or roughing it through the times of economic depression Americans have used very minimal ingredients to make meals.

In these times of extreme need Americans broughtknowledge from their home country or used whatever ingredients were cheap and plentiful to create meals to sustain them.

From these desperate times some classic recipesemerged.

Mud Apples

- 4 large apples
- A bucket of mud

Prep Time: 15 Minutes; Cook Time: 45 Minutes;

For this recipe you should really have a campfire.

Using the mud, coat your apples completely in a nice layer. Spread the coals of your fire and lay the mud coated appleson them. Build up the sides with the smoldering coals. Allow the apples to bake and the "clay" to harden around them for 45 minutes.

Be careful once they are done as you will have to remove the hardened clay shell and they will be smoking hot insideas well. Spoon the cooked apple out and enjoy!

Gorge Pasta

- 1 Cup Raw Macaroni
- 1 Can Stewed Tomatoes
- 1 lb. Cheddar Cheese

Cook Times: 15 Minutes

Cook your pasta until it is nice and tender. Drain and allowit to steam for a minute or two. Add the stewed tomatoes, cheddar cheese and hot macaroni into a bowl and stir around until the cheese is completely melted

Hot Water Cornbread

Prep Times: 5 Minutes; Cook Times: 10 Minutes

- ❖ 4 cups of boiling water
- ❖ 1 cup yellow cornmeal
- ❖ 1/4 cup flour
- ❖ 1/2 canola oil
- ❖ 1 tsp salt
- ❖ 1 Tbsp sugar (optional)

Combine the dry ingredients in a bowl. Add boiling water, and stir until you get the consistency of pancake batter. Use a wooden spoon to do the stirring.

Heat about a 1/4 inch of oil in a cast iron skillet on medium high heat. Use about a quarter cup of batter per cake. Pour the batter into you hot oil and fry the cake on both sides. Delicious with fresh honey.

Sweet Potatoes in Cream and Butter

- ❖ 6 sweet potatoes
- ❖ 1 Tbsp butter
- ❖ 1/2 cup milk
- ❖ 1/2 cup cream
- ❖ Salt and pepper
- ❖ A speck of nutmeg

Prep Times: 10 Minutes; Cook Times: 15 Minutes;

Start by peeling and dicing your sweet potatoes. Be sure to cut them all in similar sizes so they cook evenly. Place them in a pot with your milk and cream. Simmer the potatoes for about 10 minutes or until they are softened enough that a fork will pierce them without resistance. Mash them with the back of a wood spoon and add your butter and seasonings.

HOW NORTH AMERICAN INDIANS AND EARLY PIONEERS MADE PEMMICAN

"A starving man will eat with the wolf." –
Oklahoma Indians

Pemmican is a concentrated nutritionally complete food invented by the North American Plains Indians. It was originally made during the summer months from dried lean Buffalo meat and rendered fat as a way to preserve and store the meat for use when traveling and as a primary food source during the lean winter months.

When pemmican was discovered by our early Frontiersmen (explorers, hunters, trappers, and the like) it became a highly sought after commodity. The Hudson Bay Company purchased tons of pemmican from the native tribes each year to satisfy the demand. The basic unit of trade was an animal hide filled with pemmican, sealed with pure rendered fat on the seams, and weighed about 90 pounds. As long as it was kept away from moisture, heat, and direct sunlight, it would last for many years with no refrigeration or other method of preservation.

There appeared to be two types of pemmican. One was a mixture of 50% shredded dehydrated lean meat and 50% rendered fat by weight. The other mixture was similar but contained 50% rendered fat, 45% shredded dehydrated meat and 5% dried and ground berries by weight. The berries were typically Saskatoon berries which grew in abundance in the Great Plains area, and are similar to blueberries.

There is much controversy as to whether the natives included the dried berries in the pemmican they made for themselves or whether they added it only to the pemmican they sold to the Hudson Bay Company "because the White Man preferred it that way". I'm of a mind that the natives consumed it both ways. The journals from the Lewis & Clark expedition clearly state that the Indian tribes they encountered consumed some berries, fruits, and tubers as part of their diet. It seems reasonable that the inclusion of some dried berries would not be out of character for the batches of pemmican made in late summer when ripe berries were available. Berries do not appear to be a nutritional requirement and they increase the chance of spoilage, so the pemmican formula in this document is for meat and fat only, and does not include them.

Please bear in mind that pemmican is NOT a raw food, as the fat needs to be heated above 200° deg. F. in order to release it from its cellular structure and drive out the moisture. It is therefore not recommended as part of a daily RAF (Raw Animal Food) diet. However, it is a useful compromise when one is traveling, for use as emergency rations, or when otherwise high-quality raw animal foods are unavailable.

It is important that the lean meat used in pemmican be dehydrated at a temperature below 120° F., and a temperature between 100° F. and 115° F. is ideal. Temperatures above 120° F. will "cook" the meat and will severely compromise the nutritional value of the pemmican. Federal and State laws require commercial dried meat products like jerky to be raised to a temperature above 150° F. which cooks the meat to a well-done state and makes it totally unsuitable for making pemmican.

Nutritional Qualities

The nutritional qualities of pemmican are unmatched when it is properly made. It can be eaten for months or years as the only food and no nutritional deficiencies will develop. Yes, that is correct, no fruits, vegetables, grains, or dairy products are required to maintain perfect health – just properly made pemmican and water.

Vitamin C and scurvy is often brought up as a concern. Explorers, hunters, and Native Americans have demonstrated over and over that consuming raw meat or meat that was dried at a temperature below 120 deg F., as long as there is sufficient fat present to supply enough calories, will maintain perfect health and prevent or cure scurvy. Those who consume salted and preserved meats, biscuits, and other processed foods, even when lemon juice is added to their diet, will often die from scurvy or other nutritional deficiencies.

Calcium and weak bones is another concern. Due to the advertising of the dairy industry, it is believed that milk, cheese, or other dairy products are essential to maintaining good bone density. It has been shown that people eating a diet of meat and fat, where the animal consumed was allowed to eat its natural diet, (usually grass), bones developed normally and remained strong with no sign of deterioration.

For the best quality pemmican, use red meat, (deer, beef, elk, bison, etc), and the rendered fat from these same animals. The animals should be grass fed or have eaten their natural diet in the wild. DO NOT include nuts, seeds, vegetable products, vegetable oils, grains, beans, or dairy products of any kind. A small amount of well dried berries (blueberries, Saskatoon, strawberries, etc) is the only acceptable addition and should not exceed 5% by weight should you choose to include them.

Directions

Ingredients:

Equal amounts by weight of very dry red meat and rendered beef tallow. If you have one pound of dried meat then you will need one pound of rendered beef tallow, two pounds of dried red meat then two pounds of rendered beef tallow, etc.

1. Rendering the Fat

Rendering fat is a simple process and most of us are familiar with it as it is one of the end results of frying bacon. The process of frying the bacon releases the fat from the cellular structure of the meat and drives off the water. It is the boiling off of the water that actually makes bacon pop and sizzle. The fat itself just turns to a liquid.

Our goal in our rendering process is a bit different from frying bacon in that it is the fat we wish to keep rather than the crisp "cracklin's", which by the way taste good when they are still warm with a bit of salt. If you don't want them they make wonderful dog treats when cool.

> We also want to keep the ultimate temperature of the fat as low as possible. I try to keep it below 250° F. and usually shoot for a final temperature of around 240° F. You gain nothing by raising the temperature any higher than 240- 250 other than more damage to the fatty acids which we want to avoid as much as possible. In short, you need the temperature high enough to boil off the water in a reasonable length of time, but as low as practical to maintain the nutritional value and not denature the structure of the fatty acids any more than necessary.
>
> There are two generally accepted methods of rendering. One is to place the fat in a pot and heat it on the stove top. The other is to place the fat in a roasting pan and put it in the oven with the temperature set between 225° – 250° F.
>
> The stove top method can be completed in about one hour and requires constant attention. The oven method takes 12 hours or more, but can be left unattended during the entire process. I will be covering the stove top method here with comments on the oven method mixed in but not demonstrated.

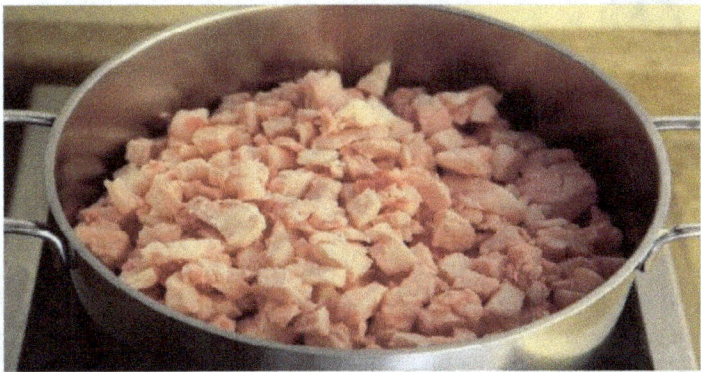

Cut the fat into small pieces about ½" square. Place the diced fat in a stock pot or pan. I select my pot size such that the raw fat fills the pot about ¾ full. This gives me head room to stir and mix without slinging fat all over the stove or counter. It also fills the pot deep enough with the liquid fat so that I can use a candy thermometer to keep track of the temperature.

If you are using the oven method just put your fat in a good sized roasting pan and pop it in the oven set between 225° to 250° F and then go away for 12 to 24 hours. The oven thermostat will take care of the temperature for you.

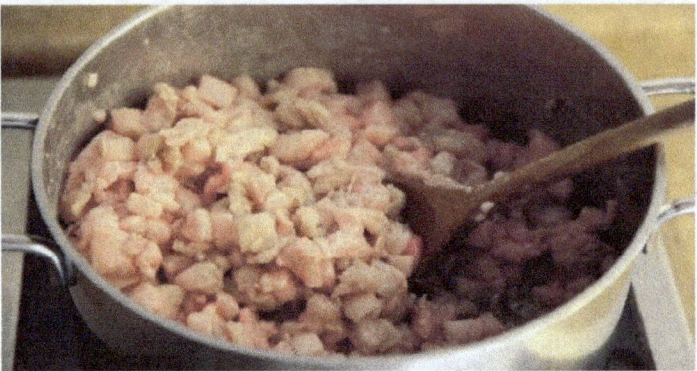

Set your burner to medium high heat and stir well about every minute or so for the first 10 minutes. This will keep the bottom from overheating while enough fat is being liberated to cover the bottom of the pan.

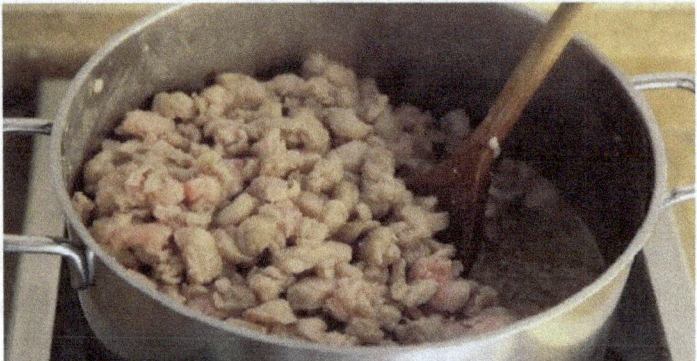

After about 10 minutes you'll see a pool of fat forming on the bottom which should be merrily boiling away. You can now rest a bit and stir every 5 minutes or so just to keep things well mixed.

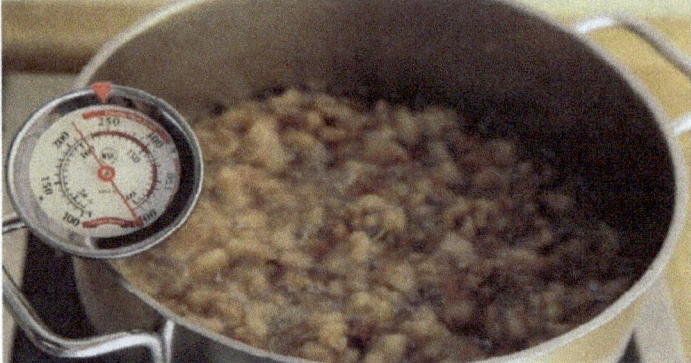

After about 30 minutes the liquid fat should be deep enough to cover all the chunks and it should have the appearance of a rolling boil. Reduce the temperature to medium heat and put a candy thermometer into the fat making sure it does not touch the bottom of the pan. The water boiling off the fat will keep the temperature around 220° F for a while, but there will come a point where the temperature will start rising.

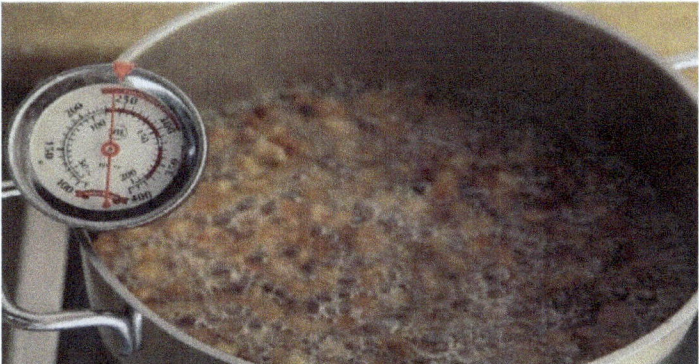

Keep stirring occasionally and keep your eye on the thermometer. As it begins to rise, lower the heat setting to keep the temperature around 230° to 240° F. The picture above is after about 45 minutes. The cracklin's are beginning to turn dark in color, the boiling is slowing down, and the temperature of the fat is rising requiring close attention to the heat setting.

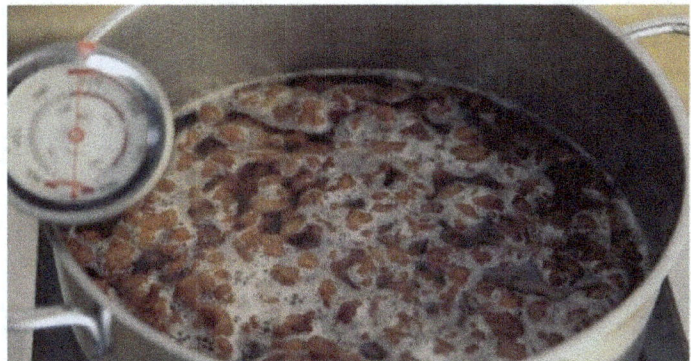

After about one hour the major boiling action will have stopped and there will just be small bubbles rising from the fat. 90% of the cracklin's will be a chestnut brown color. The lighter chunks may have a bit more fat left in them, but it is not worth the effort to extract it. If you did the oven method, the fat in your roasting pan should have a similar look.

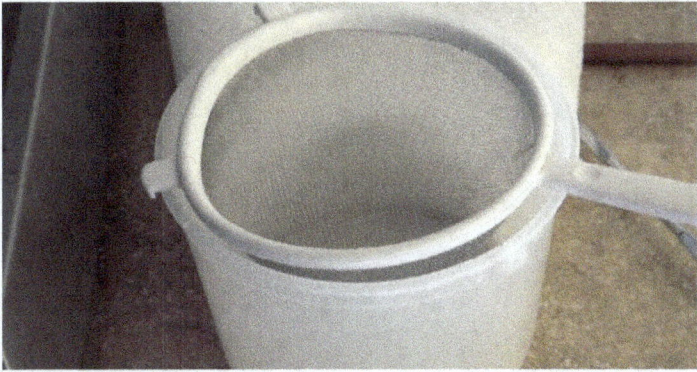

Now take a good sized strainer and place it the container where you will store your rendered fat.

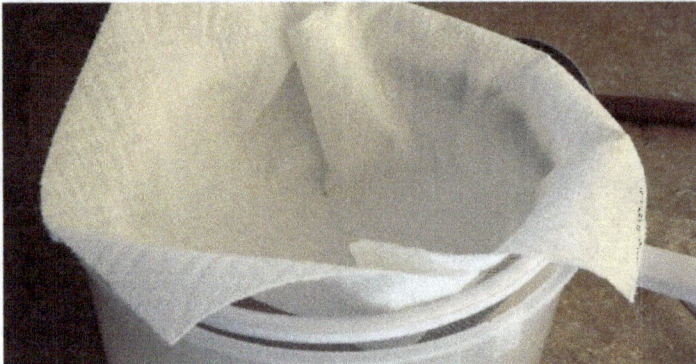

Line the strainer with a single layer of paper towel. This will filter out the sediment and just allow the liquid fat to drip through.

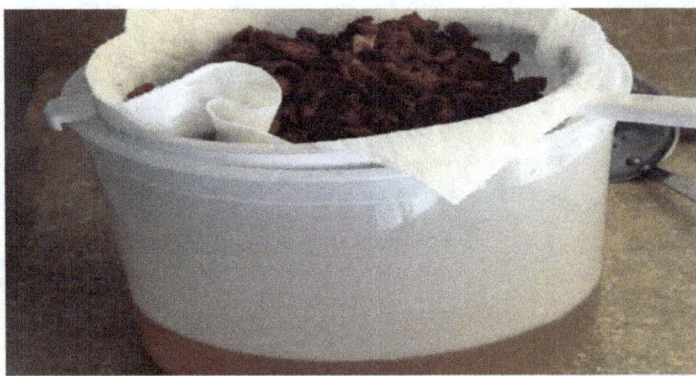

From your pot or roasting pan pour the fat, cracklin's and all, into the lined strainer. Press on the cracklin's with a serving spoon to press as much fat out of them as possible.

When you've gotten all the fat you can, remove the strainer and set the container aside to cool. You can sprinkle the cracklin's with a bit of salt and pepper and enjoy them as a snack, set them aside to cool for dog treats, or discard as you wish.

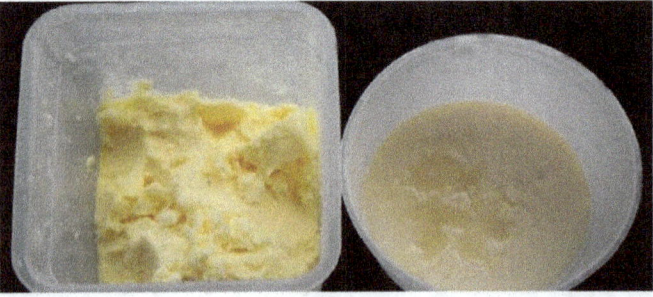

The square tub is tallow that was rendered from the fat of grass fed animals. It is a deep butter yellow from the caritinoids (the fat soluble vitamin "A" precursor that gives carrots their orange color) that gets stored in the animal's fat from the green grass they eat. The round bucket on the right is the tallow we just rendered from fat that I got from a local market. The putty color is typical of the fat rendered from grain fed animals. There is little or no carotene stored in the fat of grain fed animals.

There is also a major difference in the fatty acid profile of grain-fed vs. grass-fed animals. The grass fed animal fat is between 25 and 50 percent healthy Omega 3 fatty acids. The grain fed animal's fat is only 2 to 3 percent Omega 3. Omega 3 fatty acids are critical to the development and maintenance of our brain and nerve tissue. Overall, the meat and fat from grass fed animals has far greater nutritional value than grain fed beef. Therefore, if you want to make pemmican that meets all nutritional requirements without the need for additional supplementation, both the lean meat and the fat should come from grass fed animals.

2. Dried Meat Preparation

To make any useful amount of pemmican, a large quantity of well dehydrated lean meat is required. You can use a dehydrator or set the oven to the lowest possible temperature (around 150 degrees) and put the strips of meat directly onto the rack. Crack the oven door to prevent moisture buildup. Let the meat dry out for about fifteen hours, or until it is crispy.

Generally, well dried meat will weigh just slightly less than 1/3 of its raw weight. Therefore, 10 pounds of raw lean meat will yield about 3 lbs. of thoroughly dehydrated meat. Since pemmican is 50% fat and 50% dried meat by weight, 3 pounds of dried meat will make 6 pounds of pemmican which will be equal to about 18 pounds of fresh meat.

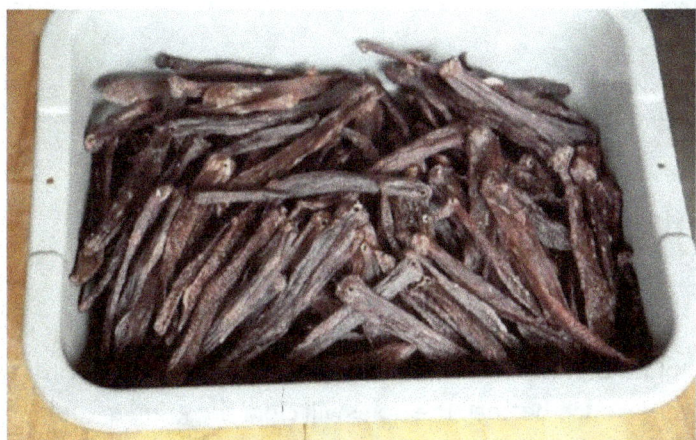

Start with well dried red meat: Beef, Bison, Deer, Elk, etc. Make sure that the strips of meat are thoroughly dry all the way through. Any observable moisture in the meat will provide an environment for mold and bacteria to grow. If the strips of meat are bent double they should crack and not be rubbery.

Traditionally the meat used for pemmican is dried without salt or any other seasoning. If you choose to season your meat I suggest that you go very lightly – less than half of what you would use for jerky. **Use only dry spices like garlic powder, pepper, cumin, chili powder, and salt etc.**

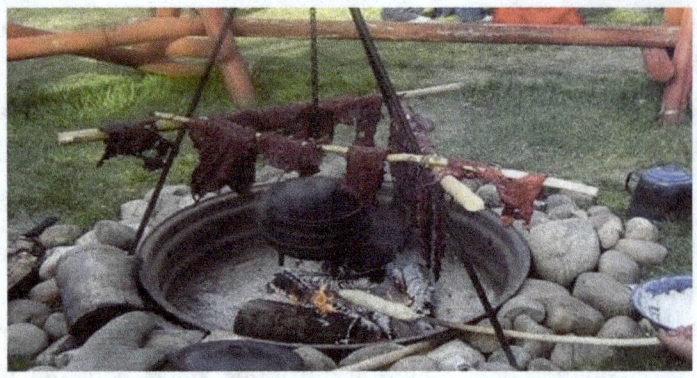

Traditional meat drying - Photo credits: John Johnston

NEVER, NEVER, NEVER make pemmican with meat that has been marinated in soy sauce, wine, or any marinade that contains sugar of any kind, and no vegetable oils of any type. I always make my pemmican without salt or seasoning and usually prefer eating it that way, but on occasion sprinkle a bit of salt or steak seasoning on it at the time I eat it for a change of pace – be careful, a little bit of seasoning goes a long way in this dense food.

Grind the meat to a fibrous consistency like a fluffy, but slightly chunky mulch. I use a meat grinder with the largest plate (biggest holes) possible. The grinder above is a large #32 manual ChopRite with a 1 ½ horsepower

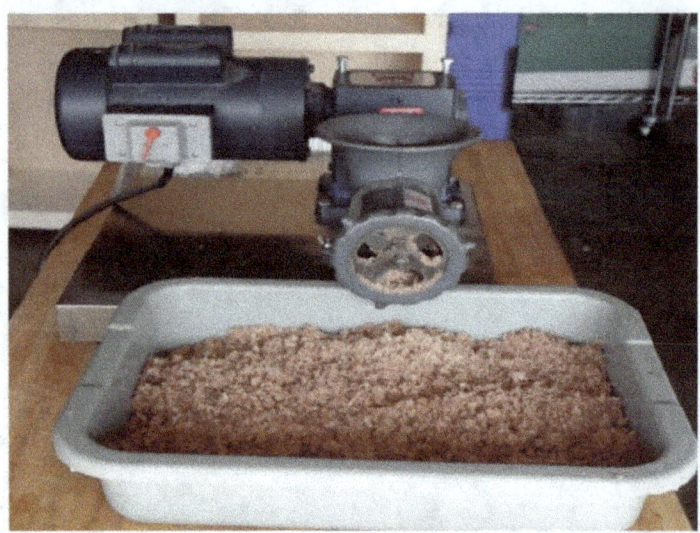

motor in place of the handle, and fitted with a "bean" plate that has 3 very large oval holes. If you attempt to use a plate with small holes, (½" may work, ¾" or larger is much better), the holes will clog, the grinder could lock-up, and you may damage it. Feed one strip at a time and wait until the exit holes begin to clear before adding the next strip. If it is too chunky and not well shredded, run it through a second time.

Alternatively you can shred the meat in a food processor using the steel blade, or in a blender. When using these options it will be helpful to chop the dried meat into smaller pieces, and some people pick up the blender and shake it while grinding to keep the un-ground chunks moving into the blades for a more even grind.

Traditionally the dry meat was pounded into a powder using rocks. I've tried the pounding method using a hammer and a small blacksmith's anvil. Unless you have a lot of time and need the exercise I don't recommend it. It is a lot of work.

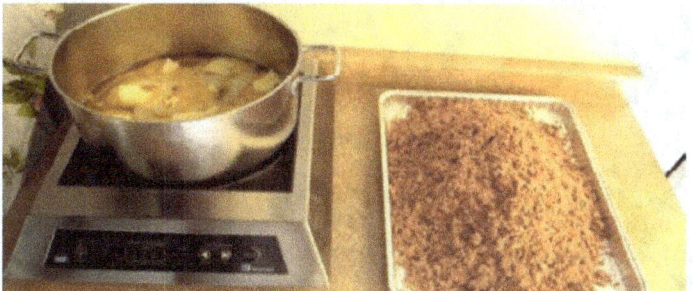

Weigh the amount of ground meat that you have and then weigh out an equal amount of rendered animal fat from the rendering process above. Fat from red meat animals is preferable for best nutrition and keeping qualities as it becomes very firm when cool – similar to candle wax. No vegetable oils or butter should be used.

Pork or lamb fat can be used but are not recommended as the fatty acid profile is different and they melt at too low a temperature. This can cause the fat and lean to separate in warm weather, so storage becomes a problem unless you are willing to pack the pemmican in liquid tight containers.

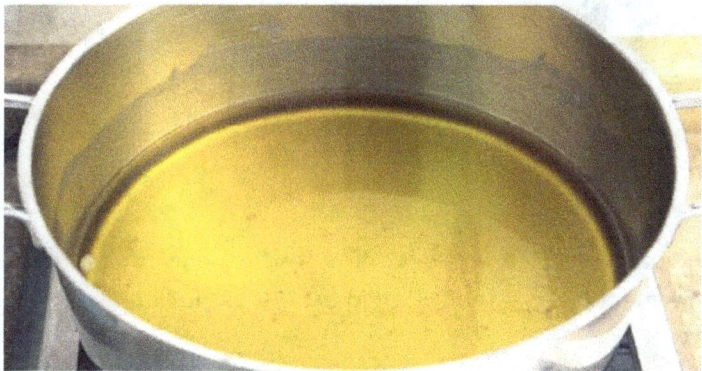

Melt the fat on low heat. It will start to melt at about 120° F.

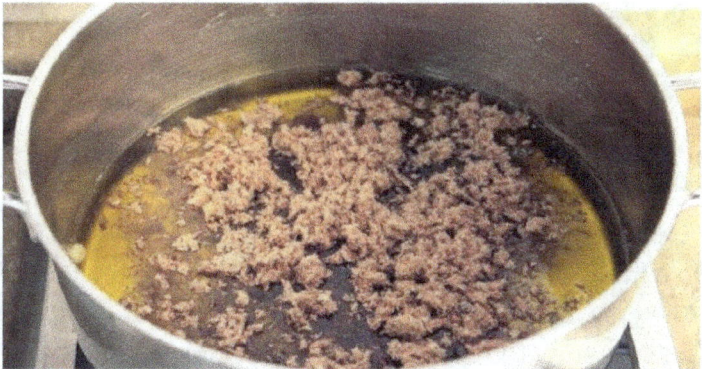

Try to keep the temperature of the fat below 150° F. You spent time drying the lean meat at low temperature to maintain its nutritional value so you don't want to deep fry it when you mix it with the fat.

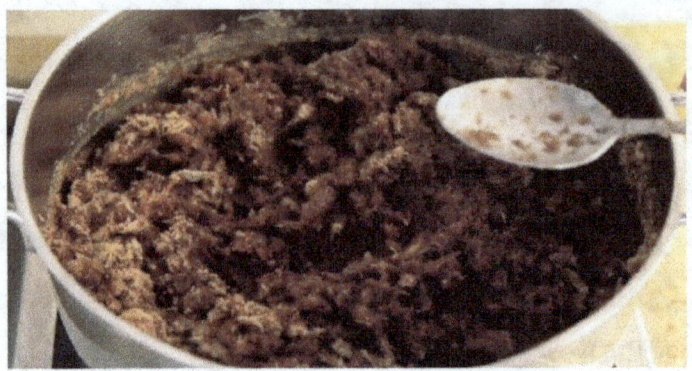

Mix the shredded meat into the melted fat and stir until well blended.

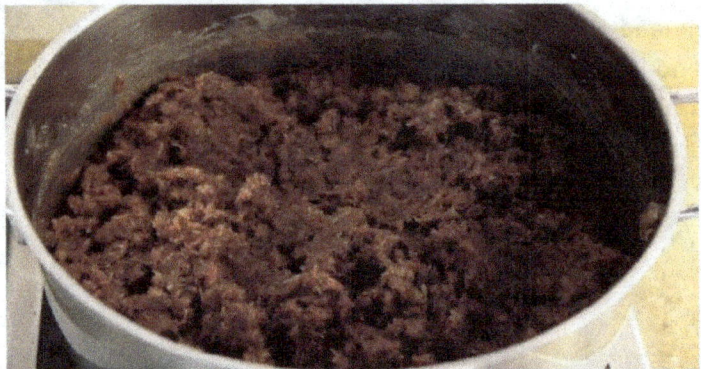

The completed mixture should look much like moist crumbled brownies. The mixture may look "wet" but most of the fat should be absorbed or coating the meat fibers – there should be little or no liquid fat pooling in the bottomof the pan.

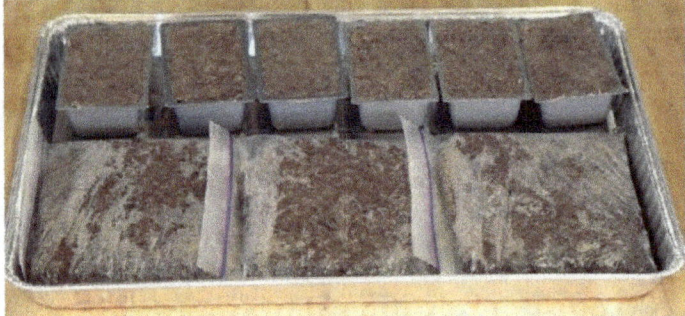

Using a sturdy spoon, press the warm mixture into a mold of your choice, or spoon into a Ziploc plastic bag and press flat, removing as much air as possible. The grey colored molds above are mini loaf pans that are slightly larger thana cube of butter and hold about 150 grams (1000 total calories) of pemmican. The Ziploc bags are sandwich sized and are loaded with about 300 grams (2000 total calories). When pressed flat they are about 5" x 6" x ½" thick. Set aside to let cool and harden. The final product will be very hard – almost like a block of wax - and will look a bit like dark oatmeal with some ground raisins stirred in.

If you are using molds such as cupcake tins or loaf pans as above, the pemmican can be removed from the mold once it is hardened and then stored in plastic bags or wrapped in a grease proof paper. One convenient method I often use is to press the mixture into lined cupcake pans and then store the resulting hockey pucks with their paper liners in gallon sized Ziploc plastic bags. Each cupcake in a standard cupcake pan will hold about 75-80 grams (around 500 calories) if you pack them solid to the top.

If you want to keep your pemmican for any length of time, it should be stored in a dark place or wrapped in light tight paper or aluminum foil as well as placed in a plastic bag to keep out air and moisture. Pemmican does not require refrigeration and can be kept for years at room temperature as long as it is kept dry, and shielded from light and direct heat.

How Much Do I Need?

One half (½) pound of pemmican per day is about the minimum required for a sedentary adult and provides about 1,500 calories. Someone doing light activities might find ¾ pound more appropriate to their needs and this would provide about 2,200 calories. Twice this amount (or more) could easily be necessary when doing hard physical labor (think digging ditches or mountain climbing).

Pemmican is the perfect food for backpacking and hiking. Ten pounds of pemmican will easily sustain a backpacker for a full week providing 1 ½ pounds of pemmican per day which would supply 4,400 calories – enough to support strenuous climbing at high altitude and in cold weather. The same 10 pounds of pemmican would supply food for two full weeks of leisure camping activities at ¾ pound per day providing 2,200 calories.

When made correctly, using grass fed lean red meat, dried at a temperature below 120°F., and rendered fat from grassfed animals, pemmican is a complete food and no other nutrients or supplements are necessary to completely meet all human nutritional requirements. No other single food is as calorie dense or nutritionally complete.

HOW THE SHERIFFS FROM THE FRONTIERS DEFENDED THEIR VILLAGES AND TOWNS

"If we desire to avoid insult, we must be able to repel it; if we desire to secure peace, one of the most powerful instruments of our rising prosperity, it must be known, that we are at all times ready for War." — George Washington

Westerns give us a vivid picture of law enforcement in the Old West. When a gang of outlaws starts to terrorize a town the frightened inhabitants beg their sheriff to do something – but usually he's either corrupt, a coward or just not up to the job. All seems lost until an enigmatic stranger appears, confronts the troublemakers and saves the day. It's a striking image – but it's wrong in almost every detail.

The people who settled the West were not shrinking violets. The fact they were out there in the first place should tell us that. These were people who'd left their homes and traveled – sometimes from the cities of the East Coast, often all the way from Europe – to make a new life in uncharted wilderness. They were pioneers and adventurers – bold, determined people. They may have lived in towns but in most cases they had built those towns themselves – few western settlements at the time had seen two generations raised there, and many were only a few years old. Even recent arrivals had struck out on a long, tough and often dangerous journey to reach their new home, and not many of them were easily scared.

Then there were the lawmen. Movies and novels often mix up the roles of marshal and sheriff, but they were very different. The history of the Old West mostly played out in territories that hadn't yet achieved statehood. That meant there were no state governments to take care of law enforcement.

The federal government's response was to send U.S. marshals into the new territories. The United States Marshals Service is the country's oldest law enforcement agency, set up in 1789 as the enforcement arm of the federal courts. Marshals were ideal for the job because they had extensive powers; they could hire local deputies or recruit a posse.

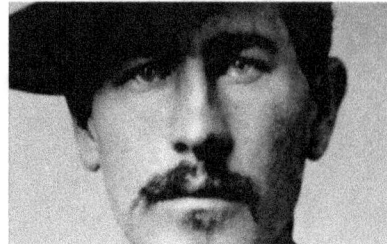

Virgil Earp was a U.S. Marshal, and he hired Wyatt Earp (picture) and Doc Holliday as assistants.

But while marshals had a lot of power there weren't many of them, certainly not enough to cover the huge and growing expanses of the West. As towns became established they started to take responsibility for their own law enforcement, in the shape of local sheriffs. The office of sheriff is an ancient one dating back to Saxon England but in the West it took on a distinctive form. Instead of an official appointed by the king these new sheriffs were elected by the townspeople, and given responsibility for law and order.

Because they were elected sheriffs tended to be trusted. There were exceptions; elections could be rigged, or enough voters bribed to elect an unpopular candidate, but in general the job was given to someone the people thought could do it. The position came with a lot of power and even more responsibility. The sheriff could appoint deputies to help him with his duties, which were many. Sheriffs often acted as tax collectors, and resolved disputes over grazing rights or access to water. They're most famous as lawmen though. In the early days, before the western territories achieved statehood, they literally had the power of life and death. A sheriff could arrest wrongdoers, hold a trial and carry out the sentence. Sometimes that meant locking a drunk up in the town jail for a few days; sometimes it meant a hanging.

Crime in the West

What sort of crime did those sheriffs have to deal with, though? Another stereotype we get from movies is that the Old West was a lawless, violent place. The truth is, in general it wasn't. In fact a typical Western town in the 1860s had a lot less crime and disorder than it does today. That's mostly down to the people who lived there and the lives they led.

The new lands of the West attracted a wide range of personalities, from visionaries who dreamed of building paradise to misfits on the run from the law or a family, but the untamed land was a ruthless judge. To survive more than a few weeks out there, never mind to successfully establish a farm or business, you had to learn to work together. Neighbors helped each other by trading supplies or lending muscle to a building project. Merchants gave credit on an honor system, and those who abused that trust soon found themselves unwelcome in town.

After the Civil War the ranks of the pioneers swelled with veterans, who brought their own camaraderie with them.

All this meant a level of trust soon developed in a Western town. People knew their neighbors, worked beside them and socialized with them. They knew they could rely on each other for help. In this atmosphere petty crime was frowned on and violence surprisingly rare.

When violence threatened it usually came from outside. There were gangs of outlaws, often made up of men who'd failed to fit in with the frontier society and banded together with others like them. As big ranchers moved in and came into conflict with small farmers they sometimes hired gangs of gunslingers to enforce their will. Later the early railway barons would resort to the same tactics. When the federal government began its war against the Plains Indians the previous good relations between settlers and the tribes broke down, and warriors began attacking farms and even small towns.

In fact the threats that faced those old-time lawmen were a lot like the ones you're likely to be dealing with in a SHTF scenario, but they're probably going to fall on you a lot quicker. After all in the West society was still being built, home by home and farm by farm. The majority of the people were part of that effort. They were used to taking care of themselves, growing their own food, digging wells for water and resolving disputes like adults.

Now imagine what it will be like when a developed society like ours, full of people who think meat grows in shrink- wrapped packages, collapses. Suddenly all those people have to fend for themselves – and unlike the old pioneers they don't have any idea how to do it. It won't be long before marauding gangs, desperate for basic necessities like food and water, are trying to take them from anyone who looks like they're managing to cope with the situation. Existing law enforcement probably won't be able to help you much, either – what elements of it haven't collapsed

will be completely overwhelmed, because chaos will spread far and fast. If you want to protect yourself, your family and your property in this scenario you're going to have to do it yourself. Many people in the USA now realize this and aim to be prepared, but a lot of them are going the wrong way about it. This is where the lessons of those old sheriffs come in.

To apply the same techniques as sheriffs in the West used, it helps to look at how your own situation resembles theirs
– and how it's different.

Equipment

Guns

The USA's high rate of gun ownership is what makes it possible to defend your community if society breaks down
– but it also increases the threat. You can bet that any group of marauders will quickly pick up ever gun they can get their hands on, while hungry refugees could also be carrying to defend themselves. Having the right guns available is going to make a huge difference to your efforts to preserve a little patch of law.

Colt still call their Single Action Army revolver – the famous Peacemaker – "The gun that won the West". It wasn't. In fact the role of handguns in the Old West has been hugely exaggerated, something else we can thank Hollywood for. Yes, many famous figures from that time carried one, but they were nowhere near as common as the movies make out. Almost every household on the frontier was armed, but guns were expensive – compared to the average income, a lot more expensive than they are now – and few people could afford a collection of them. They tended to buy one gun, and pick one that would be as versatile as possible. Usually it wasn't a revolver.

For the typical settler in one of the new American territories a handgun wasn't actually good for much. He needed a gun to put food on the table, maybe to hunt animals for their pelt, and to keep critters away from his crops. Self-defense was just something else it could be used for if necessary – few people saw that as their gun's main function – and if they did use it for protection it was more likely to be against an animal than a person. The popular image of every cowboy and rancher walking around with a six-shooter strapped to his hip simply isn't correct, as period photos show. Some did carry revolvers, but most didn't.

Rifles were far more common weapons in the West, because they could be used for hunting and had a longer range. After the Civil War there was no shortage of military-surplus rifle muskets, and many settlers carried those or similar weapons.

If there really is a gun that won the West, though, it has to be the humble 12-gauge shotgun. It's hard to imagine a more versatile workhorse firearm than this. It can be loaded with anything from a single massive projectile – ball then, slug now – to a charge of rock salt, so it's capable of bringing down most game. Anything from small birds to the largest deer can be taken with an appropriately loaded shotgun. It's also ideal for self-defense at short and medium range. No pistol cartridge comes close to the power of a 12-gauge, and loaded with buckshot it also has a much longer effective range.

Familiarity plays a part – in an emergency you'll be a lot better off with the gun you carry and use every day – but unless you've done hundreds of hours of specialist police or military handgun training, a shotgun is just an easier weapon to protect yourself with.

The same things that made a shotgun the ideal weapon in the 19th century West still hold true today – in fact, if anything its advantages have increased. There's a wider choice of ammunition than ever, including rifled slugs that are accurate and hard-hitting out to 100 yards or more. Traditional side-by-sides have been replaced with pump actions, which are extremely reliable but offer higher ammunition capacity.

Shotguns are designed for rapid, instinctive aiming, useful for hunting and a critical advantage in a self-defense situation. They also have a huge psychological effect. The sound of a pump shotgun chambering a round is instantly recognizable and highly intimidating. Cops will tell you that it often makes intruders turn tail and run without a single shot being fired. If it's SHTF time a lot of the intruders you'll be facing are starving refugees from the city. You don't want them stealing your supplies, but you don't want to shoot them either if you can avoid it.

Communications

It's amazing how quickly we've become used to today's hyper-connected world. Most of us are never out of touch, wherever we are – but only 25 years ago cell phones were a rarity and mobile internet completely unheard of. If you wanted to talk to someone while you were out you found a call box and hoped they were at home. In the Old West even that option didn't exist. There were no telephones, and the only quick way of communicating over long distances was the embryonic telegraph system. The first telegraph line went up in 1844, linking Washington, D.C. with Baltimore. By 1856 there were around 40 US telegraph companies, all based in the eastern states, but one of them
– which had recently renamed itself Western Union - had begun buying up many of the others. Western Union opened the first transcontinental line in 1861 between New York and California, and through the rest of the century the telegraph network slowly spread through the developing West.

Not every town had a telegraph station though, and few had more than one. Sending a message wasn't a fast process. Each one had to be tapped out by hand using Morse code, then written down at the receiving end. Then either the person it was addressed to had to pick it up at the telegraph station or a Western Union runner would deliver it. Even so it was a huge improvement over what went before – the Pony Express. Riders on fast horses, changing mounts frequently, could carry a 20-pound sack of mail from St. Joseph, Missouri to Sacramento, California in around ten days. The Pony Express became a legend of the West – but it closed two days after the transcontinental telegraph started operating. Still, riders were the quickest way to get a message between most towns out west until well into the 1880s unless you lived beside the railroad.

If society collapses you'll suddenly find your communication options at least as narrow as those of a 19th century pioneer. Cell phones, landline exchanges and the internet will go down quickly. The only modern communications that will work are self-contained radios with their own power sources, and if you don't have them in your SHTF kit you'll be back to using riders to carry messages outside your local area. If you don't have any horses, and have to rely on automobiles or motorbikes, that's going to use valuable fuel reserves you're probably reluctant to waste – but good communications played a big part in keeping the Old West law-abiding, and they're just as important for you.

Organization

That brings us on to the next key point – how to organize. That's something a lot of preppers seem to overlook. A big part of being ready for when the SHTF is self-reliance, and that doesn't seem to sit well with committee meetings and organizing communities to work together, but it needs to be talked about. The people who set out to build the West were also self-reliant; they had to be. But they also knew they could accomplish more by working together than they could as individuals.

One family can secure and defend their own property – but they have no control over the surrounding area, and if a large enough group of marauders attacks them they're eventually going to be overrun. A loose community of hundreds of well-prepared, self-reliant people could betaken down by a dozen bandits if they only have to deal with them one or two or five at a time.

Now imagine the same dozen robbers approaching a typical 19th century town out on the frontier. The town probably only had a couple of hundred people, and they lacked most of the advantages we have today. They had no radios, no motor vehicles and the most common firearms were double-barrel shotguns and single-shot rifle muskets. But the robbers had almost no chance, because the townspeople had an informal but effective organization to keep the peace.

The Sheriff

Frontier towns couldn't support a full-time police department; everyone was too busy taming the surrounding land and building the town itself. Even the sheriff often wasn't a full-time law enforcer. Elected from among the people, he probably had a farm or business of his own to run. There were upsides to this though. Usually there wasn't a divide between law enforcement and civilians as there often is now. The townspeople knew that the sheriff was one of their own. Most of them had voted for him; the ones who hadn't still knew who he was. There was an essential link between sheriff and people; they'd chosen him to protect them from lawbreakers, and that meant he could count on their support when he needed it.

Sheriffs could call for support in many ways, but one of their most valuable assets was simply the community itself. People talked to their neighbors, in a web of information sharing that covered the district. If someone had a problem with pilfering round their farm, pretty soon everyone else would know about it and be on the lookout. Word would soon get to the sheriff, and he'd probably take a look round the area. Any opportunist criminals would quickly see that the community was on the alert, and that had a big deterrent effect.

Deputy Sheriffs

Where deterrence didn't work the sheriff had the power to deputize people to help him. Larger towns might have full-time deputies, paid from the sheriff's share of the taxes he collected. In smaller settlements the sheriff might have a pool of men he knew he could rely on, but would only deputize them when they were needed. That's the situation you'll be in if society collapses; it's not likely your local community will be big enough to support full-time deputies.

A deputy sheriff, then and now, is a person appointed by the sheriff to carry out the sheriff's duties. They have all the powers of the sheriff himself, including investigating crimes, making arrests and detaining suspects and criminals. Traditionally a deputy is an employee of the sheriff, meaning they're paid by the sheriff and are under their command.

Posses

Because they had to be paid, the number of deputies a sheriff could employ was limited. One option was to hire them only when needed, but sometimes so much manpower was needed that it just wasn't possible to hire that many people. That's where another of the sheriff's powers came in – the right to raise a posse. This comes from the tradition of Posse Comitatus, or "power of the community", and like the office of sheriff itself it goes back to English common law.

A sheriff has the power to conscript any able-bodied man into a posse when manpower is needed. Usually that happened when a fugitive had to be captured or a large group of outlaws threatened the peace. Members of a posse didn't have all the powers of a sheriff or deputy, but they did have whatever powers the sheriff delegated to them. For example, if the posse was called out for a manhunt its members would be given the power to arrest the fugitive. Other times the right to self-defense would be enough for the task.

Bringing it up to date

So law and order in the Old West was mostly handled by sheriffs and the help they could draw on from their communities, either by appointing deputies or raising a posse. The big question is, when our own society collapses, how can you use those methods to keep yourself and the people around you safe? Is it even an appropriate way to do things?

The answer to that question has to be yes. Sheriffs, unlike most modern police forces, belong to the old tradition of policing by consent. If the people didn't like the job their sheriff was doing, when his term was up they could elect someone else. That was an important check that kept most sheriffs honest. Now, with the police increasingly politicized and remote from the people, the element of consent is gone. That doesn't matter much to a powerful government that can enforce its will through force, but what about when that government loses control? If you want to preserve safety in the aftermath the first thing you need to do is get consent, because people aren't going to accept any other form of policing.

Getting yourself elected as sheriff probably isn't realistic in a SHTF scenario. People are likely to be too worried, and too involved in looking after themselves, to feel like organizing a town hall meeting. Security is a priority, though, and it's likely to be needed sooner rather than later. That means someone has to take on the responsibility. If nobody else is doing it you're going to have

to step up, and your first task is going to be building the consent you need. If you just start patrolling the area with a gun the chances are you'll be looked at with suspicion – but with the right groundwork you'll get a much better response.

The first thing to do is speak to as many of your neighbors as you can. If you can get them all together at once, great; if not, talk to them individually. Explain that you're worried about lawlessness affecting you and them, and that you have some ideas to help prevent any issues. Some will immediately see the advantages. Others might need some convincing. Focus on these points:

- ❖ Safety in numbers. A group of people working together can achieve a lot more than the same number all doing their own thing – and that applies to security, too.
- ❖ Better awareness. Being organized means sharing information, and that means everyone gets advanced warning of any developing problems.
- ❖ Less time-consuming. If every home is 100% responsible for its own security everyone will spend a lot of time checking for intruders and standing guard. That wastes time people could use producing food and adapting to the crisis.
- ❖ Safety for singles. Families can take turns checking perimeters at night or standing guard when marauders are around. Anyone living alone can't do that. If there are older people in your area they're vulnerable, too – and local safety is only as strong as the weakest link.

When you show people that you've thought about keeping the area safe from lawbreakers, and you have a plan to do most of them are going to agree. You're not trying to take over; you just have some positive suggestions to save everyo some time and gain them some security. What you'll probably find is that your friends and neighbors have been worryi about exactly those issues. Most of us think we can protect our homes by ourselves, and most of the time we can – b when a dozen armed and desperate people could raid your food supplies at any time we start to realize that we need sleep sometimes, and that leaves a lot of hours when we're not ready to respond. Ask anyone who's done time in t military how exhausting sentry duty gets – it's educational.

Once the majority of your neighbors have accepted your plan, you're ready to get started. Without announcing it you' basically got yourself elected as sheriff. Don't get carried away, but now you need to start putting the plan into effect – a that means you're going to need deputies.

This looks like the tricky bit; you have to persuade people to give up some of their time to help you out. Actually it's not th hard, though, because they'll see the benefits pretty quickly. In exchange for taking turns at patrolling the area they'll able to sleep soundly every other night, knowing that someone's out there keeping an eye on things – and ready to raise t alarm if necessary.

Showing the Flag

One of the most important things you can do is have a visible presence round the clock. That's one of the main reasons old-time sheriff would take on deputies. Many crimes are a lot easier to commit at night, but if the area's being patroll that's a big deterrent. Obviously you can't do it all yourself – you need to sleep too, and you have other things to attend So find a few volunteers who can see the benefits, and organize a shift system. These will do the job of your deputies.

How you patrol will depend a lot on the area. If it's suburban – even urban – you might need to control access. A sm neighborhood can be held together even in a major collapse, but not if refugees and raiders have easy access. Then aga you can't mobilize enough manpower to cover every road. Consider barricading most of them, at least well enough to ke vehicles out, and having checkpoints to control the one or two you leave open. A roving deputy can check the others on rounds to make sure nobody's trying to reopen them.

In a rural community homes are likely to be a lot more scattered and distances will be longer. Vehicle patrols are an opti here, as long as fuel lasts, but out of town you're more likely to have access to horses and people who can ride. They're natural choice for the job.

Anyone who's patrolling should be armed – with at least a handgun, and ideally a shotgun or rifle – and at night they'll ne a flashlight. If you have radios they should take one of those too. What you don't want is to have them fully kitted out w military-style tactical gear. They're just guys out looking after their area and their neighbors, after all. They just have to visible enough to be noticed.

Especially during the day, your deputies should be well known and approachable people. One of the most important thir they can do, apart from just being seen, is to talk to everyone they meet. That makes people feel involved in protecti themselves, which means they'll be more supportive of what you're doing. It also helps information flow around, and tha vital. Remember – most of the modern ways of passing on information will be gone, and just like in the Old West it's going to be done by face to face conversations. That's another reason for avoiding the military look – it's just psychologica harder to talk to someone who looks ready to fight a war, even if you know them. In the actual military a lot of soldie those whose job it is to talk to the locals, will walk around with no helmet or armor, and just a sidearm, even in a high thre environment. They take a risk – and break the rules – because people are more likely to tell them stuff.

of any issues that are developing. If someone's started drinking heavily, getting aggressive with family or neighbors, possibly even thinking of suicide – you'll get to hear about it, and you can keep an eye on the situation before it gets out of control.

You and your deputies have other things to do, too. You'll know the places in the area where bandits or refugees might hide up. Check them regularly for signs that anyone's been using them. Also take a look at anything that could endanger the community. If there's a levee nearby make sure it's visited daily – more often in heavy rain. Make sure nobody's playing around with local industries that use hazardous chemicals, and check for evidence of tampering with the water supply.

One of the likeliest challenges you'll face is groups of refugees looking for food, shelter and security. You can't take them in; your own resources, no matter how well prepared you are, will be stretched enough as the crisis goes on. Be firm, but compassionate. You need to turn them away but don't use force unless they do it first. They're Americans, after all, and they're not to blame for what's happened. Some of them might even have been prepared for a social breakdown but had to move out because their home was threatened or destroyed. Give them what help you can without eating into your own reserves – directions to safe areas, even some medical supplies for anyone who's really sick or injured.

Eventually news is going to spread that your community has managed to hold itself together, and no matter how small it is – even if it's just you and one or two neighbors – someone's going to think of trying to take your resources away from you. There's a good chance that when they see you're prepared and vigilant they'll back off and look for an easier target – but they might not. That's the worst case scenario, and you need to be prepared for it.

Raising a posse

When you see a posse in the movies it's usually been raised to pursue a fugitive. That was certainly one of their functions, but not one you're likely to be calling on. Your priority is to keep wrongdoers out of your community. If they run it's usually best to just let them get away – chasing them uses manpower and resources you can't afford. But posses had another use, and that was for self-defense against a large group of attackers. That's something you're almost certainly going to need.

Sheriffs in the Old West had a legal right to draft manpower, backed up by the threat of penalties under Posse comitatus. That's an advantage you won't have. Law will have broken down; you're trying to hold a little piece of it together, but you can't do it by imposing fines on people who won't join your posse. Ten to one they aren't going to pay the fines, either. You'll have to use persuasion – and, again, most people will see the sense behind it. Those who don't will probably change their minds the first time your posse proves its worth.

Raising a posse isn't something you can leave until the barbarians are at the gates. You have to know who you can call on who'll be willing to help. Traditionally that was all able-bodied men; now it's any able-bodied adult. You have to make sure they all have access to a gun, ideally a long gun. If any don't, see if you can get those with multiple guns to loan one – and make sure the borrower knows how to use it. Arrange a place for the posse to assemble if gunfire breaks out; somewhere central and easily reached, but not in the line of fire from the ways into your neighborhood. If you can, and you have enough people, organize them into teams and try to spread any veterans among those teams to stiffen them.

When the community comes under attack the last thing you want is for everyone to rush towards the sound of the guns. What if the raiders have split into two groups? Keep a reserve to deal with anything unexpected. An old sheriff wouldn't take everyone with him; he'd leave at least one trusted deputy and enough men to protect the town while he was gone.

Sheriffs in the Old West had some other powers that you don't. They could convict, and imprison or hang, lawbreakers. Don't even go there unless it's clear the disaster is permanent. Yes, you could lock someone up in your garage and call it the town jail, but you'd just have to feed them. As for executions, that's very dangerous territory. Even in the worst case scenario, like a major EMP attack, there's a good chance the government will regain control eventually. If that happens you don't need

questions being asked about what happened during the crisis. The same goes for lynchings; if you're the one who maintained the law – even unofficially - and a criminal was lynched, you're going to carry the can for it. When raiders arrive, aim to drive them off. If any get shot in the process that's legitimate self-defense, but frontier justice is a different story.

Law enforcement in the Old West was all about the community looking after itself. It was based on consent, on power exercised by a sheriff chosen from among the people. That's the way the law should be maintained, and many of today's social problems trace back to the fact that it isn't done that way anymore.

After the SHTF[4] it's going to be different – surviving communities will have to return to the ways of the Western pioneers, because there will be no other way to maintain law and order. If those communities don't adopt the Western way of keeping the peace then they won't last; however strong and self-reliant they are they'll inevitably be overwhelmed, one house at a time, by those who emerge from the wreckage all around them. The traditions of the sheriff, America's iconic lawman, were essential to building this country. They'll be just as essential to rebuilding it after a collapse.

---

[4] SHTF is an acronym (Shit Hits the Fan), meaning a very serious disaster situation, economic crisis, EMP, etc

SPYCRAFT
MILITARY CORRESPONDENCE DURING THE 1700S TO 1900S

"The two words 'information' and 'communication' are often used interchangeably, but they signify quite different things. Information is giving out; communication is getting through." - Sydney J Harris

During the American Revolutionary War in the 1700s and the Civil War in the 1800s, technology was not as advanced as it is today. Confidential messages and top secret information had to go by word of mouth or ciphered documents. Spycraft was a must and certain skills were required in an effort to protect vital messages that could end the war. Connections, networks, relationships, and knowledge were required of potential spies. They played an important role in carrying and delivering information as it decided what the next move would be and how they would carry it out. Thus, different methods were developed to protect the messages in case they were intercepted.

Rectal Acorn, Silver Ball, and Quill Letters

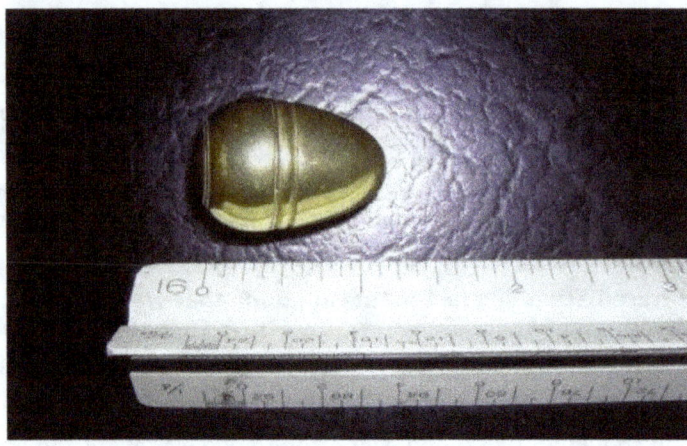

(The Rectal Acorn, courtesy of the Museum of Confederacy)

In 2009 a woman whose ancestor was a Confederate in the American Civil War visited the Museum of Confederacy with an acorn-shaped object in her hand. It was a little over an inch long and was made of brass. There were no inscriptions or markings on it. She told the museum that it was a device that her ancestor had used to carry, protect, and deliver secret messages to destinations both near and far. According to stories passed down to her by her family, spies would encapsulate the message in the acorn and hide it in their rectum until they reached the assigned place where the message was to be delivered. Only then could they push the acorn-like container out.

Similar to the rectal acorn, a silver ball was also used to hide information vital to their cause. Small, folded papers with the message were carefully placed in the ball. Because it is as small as a musket bullet, it could

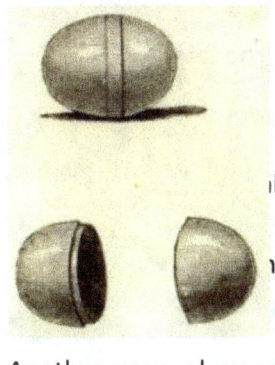

One particular unlucky spy was Daniel Taylor. He was tasked to carry a message from British General Henry Clinton to John Burgoyne. Once he realized that he was going to be caught and forced to give the message, Taylor swallowed the ball hurriedly. However, adding salt to injury, the ⟨...⟩ him swallow something, which prompted them to force him to drink an emetic that ⟨...⟩ out of his stomach. In an impressive display of will, Taylor grabbed the ball and ⟨...⟩ fortunately, when threatened with having his gut sliced open, he agreed to a second ⟨...⟩ and chose to save his life temporarily. He was later executed for treason.

Another unusual way to hide messages was to use the tight hollows of quills made from goose feathers. Because quills were a common medium for writing, it reduced suspicion, detection, and risk. Messages were written in thin strips of paper that could be rolled up to fit in the small hollow. The goal was that the spy could easily discard the message in worst-case scenarios, like Daniel Taylor.

One message written by Henry Clinton during the revolutionary war was preserved in the Collections of the Clements Library. It was a particularly long message so they had to cut it into two parts to insert it in the quill easier.

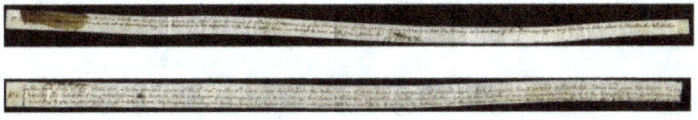

(Both images from the Collections of the Clements Library)

Invisible Ink

The different forms of hiding messages listed above may be something you've never heard of, and if you have, it might have been from museum tours or history classes. The invisible ink method could be something you're more familiar with. Today, there are different kinds of pens that can produce the same effect as the ones our ancestors used. Some pens are equipped with clear ink that could only be seen once subjected to UV light. Our ancestors had no such luxury. What they had was the basics: ferrous sulfate, water, and paper.

The "ink" was composed of ferrous sulfate mixed with water. During the war, a popular strategy was to disguise the actual message in between the lines of an innocent letter that was written with normal ink. Using the mix that makes the invisible ink, soldiers, spies, and generals wrote on the original, non-threatening letter. The recipients of the message could reveal the content of the letter written with the invisible ink by subjecting the paper to heat or a chemical reagent like sodium carbonate.

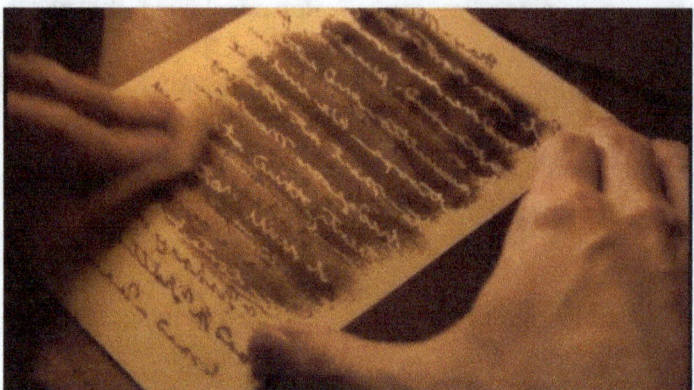

It was the preferred strategy because as George Washington said during the Revolutionary War, it reduced the risk of detection and interception which meant that ultimately, it could save a courier's life. The invisible ink was known as the sympathetic stain and Washington's agents utilized its full potential in acquiring intelligence about the movements, inventory, and plans of the other side. He instructed his people to use any type of paper, such as that used in pocketbooks, receipts, encyclopedias, and just about any kind of publication or book of small value.

Today, invisible ink is available on the market in different forms. It could come as a stylus, a pen, or a marker. However, the reality is, not everybody is willing to spend their extra dollars on a pen. Even more so, in an apocalypse, not everyone will be equipped with it, but in such a scenario, having one could be vital in survival. Luckily,

anyone can make invisible ink with almost the most basic items found in anyone's kitchen or home.

All you need to have is the most important ingredient: lemons. A scientific explanation for this would be the fact that lemons contain carbon compounds that are colorless at room temperature and become more distinct when treated to heat as it releases the carbon, making the substance darker. The recipe is easy and actually fun to try.Besides, you could always make lemonade or a lemon- based sauce with the excess.

The ingredients you're going to need are the following:

- ❖ Half of a lemon
- ❖ One half teaspoon of water
- ❖ Small bowl or any container
- ❖ Spoon
- ❖ Any kind of paper that you can write on
- ❖ Q-tips/toothpick/inkless pen/paintbrush
- ❖ A lamp with a hot lightbulb or a candle

The procedure is as follows:

- ❖ Squeeze the lemon in your container.
- ❖ Add the water, and stir throughly.
- ❖ Dip your Q-tip (or whatever you're using to write) into the mixture.
- ❖ Write your message on a piece of paper. You couldwrite a decoy message first using a pencil or a pen to make it fun.
- ❖ Let it dry. Your message will become colorless onceit dries.
- ❖ To reveal the message, hold the paper over the lightbulb or a flame (be careful not to burn the paper or yourself).

An alternative that can be used is milk. All you need is to dip your Q-tip into the milk, write the message on your paper, and let it dry for at least 30 minutes. Your message will appear if you expose it to heat.

If however, you don't have lemons or milk in your home, you can still make an invisible message by using two sheetsof paper with one of them preferably blank. Place the blankpaper under the one you're going to write on. Using a pen or pencil or anything that could put pressure, write your message on the top paper. The recipient of your message only needs to gently shade over the bottom paper to view the content.

Mask Letters

A more complicated type of hidden message is the mask letter. It was mostly the British that utilized this technique during the Revolutionary War. It was known to them as theCardan system, named after Geronimo Caradano who wasone of the most famous code-makers at that time. The mask letters required a lot of skill, patience, and intelligence. Because it was meant to be read through a mask or a shaped, cutout template, the writer had to compose a decoy message around the secret message.

Another necessary step that the British took when they used the mask letters was to send the letter through a different route than the mask. It could be that there were separate couriers for both the letter and the mask. It was imperative that the mask and the letter went in different ways so that if the letter was intercepted, it would just be an innocent letter stating general facts or exaggeratinggood news.

The Clements Library was able to preserve one of the maskletters that Henry Clinton sent to John Burgoyne. It is likelythat make everything easier, Clinton must have written the secret message before adding words and sentences to create a lett that makes sense if read without a mask. Thecontent of the letter was mainly to inform Burgoyne of theirmilitary success without making anything obvious. Once placed under the mask, his real message appeared, which revealed a completely different content. The actual letters were preserved in the Clements Library.

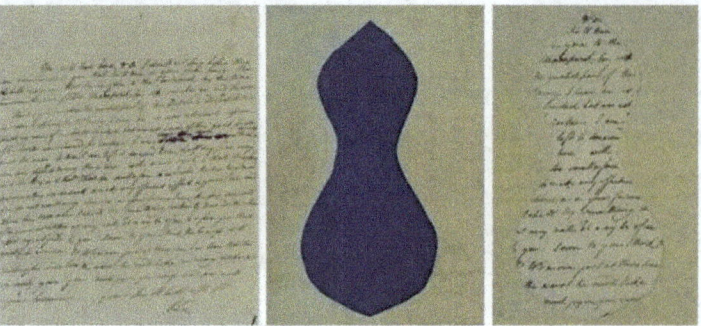

(From the collections of the Clements Library)

Despite the big names and history attached to the mask letter, it's still a secret writing technique that anyone can make today. Here's how:

Materials:

- Blank paper
- Cardboard/Paper (it's okay if it has print)
- Pen
- Envelope (Optional)

Procedure:

- Cut out your chosen shape of the mask on the cardboard.
- Place the mask over the blank paper.
- Write your secret message within the mask.
- Remove the mask and make sure that it is readable.
- Fill the paper with words or sentences to hide your secret message. (Note: The content must be innocent and must not give away your secret message.)
- Put the letter in the envelope and address it to your recipient.
- Send your letter!

During the 1700s and the 1800s spycraft required a huge amount of skill and scientific knowledge for the different methods to succeed. Resources were limited and they had to utilize whatever was within reach to create effective ways of carrying and delivering information. A strong will and determination were necessary to carry the message.

Today, we have access to advanced technology and even greater knowledge. In the past, invisible ink was created with tannic acid. Now, all we need is a lemon or a carton of milk and even e-mails can be encoded. Protecting yourself is easy when you have the money. But again, in worstcase scenarios like an EMP, communication will be so rudimentary and information will be so powerful that whoever possesses it will be king!

WILD WEST GUNS FOR SHTF AND A GUIDE TO ROLLING YOUR OWN AMMO

- By Mike Searson -

"The rifle itself has no moral stature, since it has no will of its own. Naturally, it may be used by evil men for evil purposes, but there are more good men than evil, and while the latter cannot be persuaded to the path of righteousness by propaganda, they can certainly be corrected by good men with rifles." —
Jeff Cooper

A true end of the world scenario, with no electricity, power or other conveniences could very well transform us into users of 19th century technology. How likely this scenario could happen is a matter of opinion, but it is something that should give us a reason to prepare.

Modern Firearms

Most preppers and survivalists are familiar with the modern standby firearms: Glock, SIG, AR, AK, shotgun, etc. We love them too and always have a few of each on hand, but an unimaginable disaster could render them obsolete rather quickly. A high end semiauto is a thing of beauty with a stockpile of ammo and the skill in knowing how to use it, but what happens when a part breaks and the factory and all its suppliers are gone?

An amateur gun smith can make almost any part within reason, but we like to keep a few of the older and more reliable guns that use fewer moving parts and can be repaired at a pre-industrial revolution level of technology and tools.

Handguns

One of our favorites in this category is the Ruger Blackhawk line of revolvers.

The Blackhawk was the first major successful clone of Colt's legendary 1873 Single Action Army revolver, aka the "Peacemaker". The revolver in the picture was issued to the US Cavalry early in 1874. (Photo credits: Hmaag). Ruger went with a single piece frame and used modern steel and aluminum in the manufacturing process to build a much stronger revolver than anything Colt ever turned out. In 1977 they introduced the transfer bar in

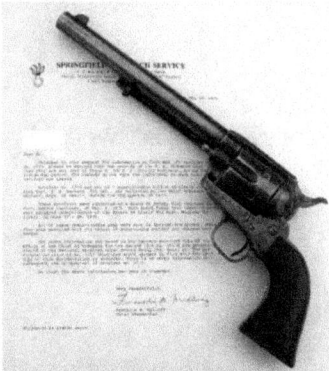

order to make it safe to carry six rounds as opposed to five in the cylinder.

Other improvements included useable adjustable sights and an ability to mount a scope or electronic sight on the revolver. Admittedly, they do not have the graceful flowing lines of the classic SAA. If you think you need that "look" there is a line called the Vaquero that uses fixed sights, but is otherwise the same handgun, although this should not be confused with the "New Vaquero" built on a slightly smaller frame.

A Blackhawk, Super Blackhawk or Vaquero (original or "Old Model" not the "New Vaquero") in 45 Colt can be loaded to pressures exceeding the modern 44 Magnum. Thus it is capable of taking any game in North America and is effective against two-legged predators as well. These single action revolvers epitomize strength and will outlive generations of shooters. Their simple design means they will outperform modern double action revolvers in the maintenance department whose lock work is more suited to a watchmaker than an amateur gunsmith, too.

They may not have the capacity or ability to reload quickly, but this can be remedied by carrying a pair of them and remembering the "Gunfighter's Motto" of the fastest reload being a second gun.

Rifles

When it comes to a rifle that you want to be able to rely on, you may want to consider a quality single shot chambered in 45-70. We chose this cartridge for its range, power level and like the straight wall revolvers we talked about, it is quite easy to reload.

The Ruger Number One, Thompson Center line of single shots and even the reproduction Sharps rifles from Pedersoli, Cimarron and others make great candidates.

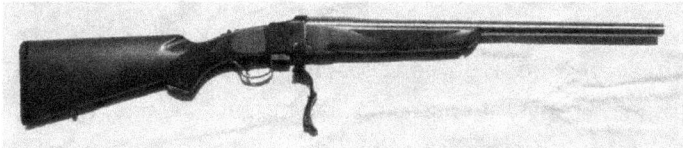

(Ruger No. 1 single-shot with custom barrel with action open – photocredits Arthurrh)

As in the case with the semi auto handguns, we are not saying to discard your modern equipment, but having a few "Old Tech" designs on hand is just a safe bet.

Ammunition

As has been witnessed in the first half of the year 2013 firearms can become useless without a steady supply of ammunition. It does not take an act of war, alien invasion, zombie apocalypse, Congressional writ or Executive Order to halt the ammunition supply; the market can easily suffer as a result of speculation and panic buying.

When big box discount stores have to limit customer's purchases to 2 boxes a day it is a pretty good indication that it has gone beyond the warning stage.

Most shooters and those with a preparedness mindset could see events like these coming months if not years in advance and built their supply steadily. However, it was noticed that as the supply situation did not resolve within a reasonable amount of time, these prepared shooters had to resort to using ammunition that was saved for a rainy day with no signs for replenishment in sight.

Even dedicated reloaders of ammunition faced the same pitfalls as the companies who make ammunition also make reloading components. The major manufacturers saw their components going right back to their own production lines to feed the consumer demand for more ammunition.

When traditional methods of acquiring ammunition are not available, the shooter needs to think outside the box on occasion in order to ensure that their ammunition supply stays constant. With regard to reloading ammunition and casting or swaging bullets, it is essential to take every reasonable precaution suggested by the manufacturers involved. There is always an inherent danger involved, but this can be strongly minimized by practicing safe loading and handling procedures.

Again, we can look to the time of the Old West, when the art of reloading was born, but take advantages of modern machinery and methods at the same time. During our frontier days, reloading or even casting bullets was more often than not a necessity. Most black powder firearms came with a bullet mold to cast the appropriate sized bullet and prior to the era of cartridge firearms, powder was carried in metal flasks or powder horns.

Reloading Components

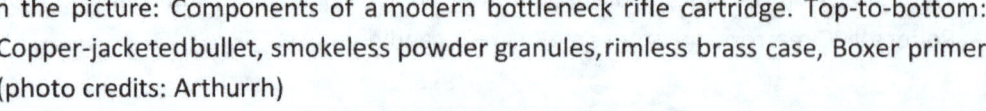

In the picture: Components of a modern bottleneck rifle cartridge. Top-to-bottom: Copper-jacketed bullet, smokeless powder granules, rimless brass case, Boxer primer (photo credits: Arthurrh)

If you were to read an article or a book on hand loading published in the past 100 years, the one statement that is constantly parroted is the great "savings" that comes with reloading. However, if the cost of brass, bullets, primers and powder was tabulated; this savings comes across as minimal, especially when factoring in the cost of dies, presses and other equipment. Over a long period of time the savings becomes more

apparent, particularly when reloading the same cases repeatedly. As a business plan, many potential ammunition manufacturers have failed, even when purchasing components at wholesale or distributor prices. What is it that makes hand loading profitable or even preferable to reselling another manufacturer's ammunition?

The answer is in sourcing the components. We determined long ago that sourcing one or two components independently was the key to making a reloading business profitable, but this mentality can be applied to the shooter looking to produce their own ammunition.

The manufacture of modern primers and smokeless powder should not be attempted by the novice and should be handled by companies that adhere to strict quality control. For our purposes that leaves brass cases and bullets.

The Cartridge Case

Sourcing cartridge cases is the basic foundation of a reloading effort. It starts with the shooter saving their cases and perhaps obtaining cases from other sources. Without brass cases, there can be no ammunition.

Most cartridge cases are made of brass, although lacquered steel, zinc, aluminum, copper and even plastic can be used. Of all these materials, only brass cartridge cases are suitable for reloading.

Brass cartridge cases can be bought in wholesale lots, bartered for or collected from shooting ranges. When using range pickups, the hand loader needs to inspect for Berdan primers. This is an older type of primer mostly found in surplus ammunition from Europe and are evidenced by two flash holes inside the case as opposed to the single flash hole of the Boxer primer. Although technically they can be reloaded, they require specialized and expensive tooling todo so, as well as a supply of Berdan primers.

Additionally steel and aluminum cases cannot be reloaded and can cause damage to the shooter's reloading equipment if this is attempted. Aluminum cases mostly have a flat grey metallic color and are most commonly found with a "CCI Blazer" head stamp on the rim of the case. They can further be identified by their use of Berdan primers and their distinctive pair of flash holes inside the case. Steel cases typically have a dark green, black or even copper colored case to reflect an anti-corrosive coating on their exterior. Like aluminum cases they are most often found with Berdan primers.

Lastly, certain calibers will only sustain a certain amount of reloading depending on the firearm that has fired them. This is most notable in 40 S&W rounds fired in pistols with unsupported chambers (1st and 2nd Generation Glocks) or 223 or 308 ammunition fired from H&K or CETME rifles which use a fluted chamber to aid in extraction. These particular pieces of brass should be avoided at all costs and make good candidates for the scrap bucket as repeatedly resizing them will weaken the brass and will eventually result in catastrophic failure.

Processing Brass Cartridge Cases

In order to be an effective hand loader, one must inspect, sort and process the brass cases in order to ensure that the ammunition will be safe to load. Processing helps eliminate the Berdan primed cases, aluminum cases, steel cases and hopefully any cases of the incorrect caliber or that are not in their correct specifications.

While inspecting cases, the shooter should look for cracks in the neck and excessive bulges near the base. More than likely these cases will not resize properly and will need to be discarded to the scrap bucket.

When using brass that has been fired and collected from a shooting range it is advisable to clean and lube the cases. This can be done in a media tumbler with crushed walnut shell or dried corncob. Polishing chemicals can be added to speed up the process as well as special lubricants that will reduce wear and tear on the reloading equipment.

Depending on the equipment used, the brass can be de- primed at this time. This is usually done via a single stage reloading press and a de-capping pin. This step in the process resizes the case mouth as well.

Primer Pocket

The primer pocket is the part of the cartridge case where the primer is seated. Some types of military surplus brass will have an extra crimp to hold the primer in place. While processing brass for reloading, the crimp will need to be removed. In extreme cases the pocket will need to be de- burred or reamed so a new primer can be seated.

Bullets and Projectiles

Bullets are the one component that can most easily be made and stockpiled by any shooter of any skill level. Again, the prospective hand loader has choices instead of simply buying bullets or even the base material with which to cast them.

When it comes to store-bought bullets, the possibilities are seemingly endless. Leafing through a supplier's catalog or scrolling through a manufacturer's webpage can be overwhelming when it comes to choosing the correct bullet for a reloading project. Most manufacturers will list the weight of the bullet (typically in grains) and the profile of the bullet as well as the composition.

With the exception of specialty made bullets, most will be sold at a similar price point. The major cost will usually be the shipping charges (bullets in bulk can be heavy). An alternative to ordering from manufacturers, distributors or internet retailers that require shipping to the customer can be in the form of finding a local bullet manufacturer where the bullets can be picked up locally. If this does not seem to be an option, the enterprising hand loader can always make bullets at home

The Cast Lead Bullet

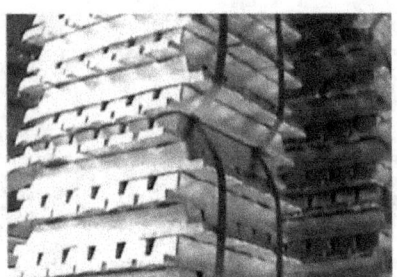

The easiest type of bullet to make is the cast lead bullet. Lead bullets work best in handgun calibers (particularly revolvers) and rifle rounds loaded less than 1000 feet per second. Any bullet travelling faster than this will cause excessive leading in the barrel. This can be alleviated in certain calibers to a degree by using a gas check; which is a cup or disc made of a harder metal that is situated at the rear of the projectile.

Lead can be bought in lead ingots of the proper alloy for shooting or it can be found by digging up the berms of shooting areas; sourced from rivers, lakes and streams in the form of old fishing sinkers or dive belts and obtained from tire shops in the form of old wheel weights. Most tire shops will be happy to give it away as they typically pay for disposal.

When lead known as bullet alloy is acquired it is actually a mixture of lead, tin and antimony. These additional elements aid in making the bullet harder than lead, by itself to reduce leaving lead deposits in the rifling of the barrel when a bullet is fired at a velocity greater than 1,000 feet per second. Recycled lead will not often have these properties.

Casting Bullets

Making cast bullets is simple in theory. The lead must be melted and poured into appropriate size molds for the caliber in question. However, lead is a toxic substance and must be handled and prepared carefully. With proper precautions this can be performed safely.

There are three essential pieces of equipment needed to cast bullets:

- ❖ Bullet mold
- ❖ Lead melting pot
- ❖ Ladle

Other equipment to have on hand includes a respirator, work gloves and an old metal spoon.

The Bullet Mold

It is paramount to research which bullet profile will work best in the firearm in question before investing in a mold. This can most easily be accomplished by the shooter purchasing factory ammunition with a lead projectile of a similar profile and trying it out in the firearm beforehand.

After determining which rounds work well, the goal will be to attempt to reproduce that load; the first step toward that goal will be to produce the bullet in question with the appropriate sized mold.

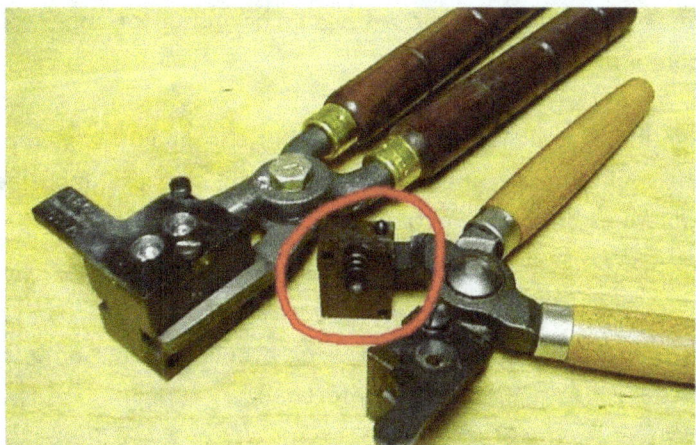

(Two bullet molds. The single cavity mold is open and empty. The double cavity mold is closed and contains two bullets – Photo Credits: Thewellman)

Bullet molds can be purchased for almost any caliber and different manufacturers will offer different patterns or profiles of different weights for each.

The Lead Melting Pot

A melting pot can be made using an old stock pot or cast iron pot. If the bullet caster has the means, a special purpose electric pot specifically made for melting lead can be purchased.

Lead melts at 600 to 621 degrees Fahrenheit. This means that the caster must be able to supply a heat source of that temperature. Because of the potential toxic fumes, the lead must be melted in a well-ventilated area, preferably outdoors. If the temperature gets hotter than 650 degrees, the potential for toxic fumes becomes even greater so a gauge of some type should be used to monitor this. The special purpose lead melting pots often have these gauges built in.

It is strongly advised to use a respirator and gloves while melting the lead.

The Ladle

The dipper or ladle is used to pour the molten lead from the pot into the mold. Some of the special purpose melting pots have a bottom spout to alleviate this. Some old time bullet casters prefer the ladle, even when they have a bottom spout because they believe the pour is more consistent.

The Melting Process

It can take 10 to 20 minutes for the lead to melt at the proper temperature.

If the caster is utilizing recycled lead, impurities will separate and rise to the surface. This will be in the form of dirt or even residual jacket material or lube with regard to recycled bullets. Recycled wheel weights may have rubber or other metal as a residue. The rubber and lube will burn off, but the metals and dirt will need to be sifted and removed from the lead pot before pouring it to cast by use of a metal spoon. These impurities will appear blackish in color and after removal may leave a trace color within the molten lead. These impurities should be placed in a metal container for disposal.

Wax shavings can be introduced to aid in fluxing out any remaining impurities. After stirring in the wax, the caster should scrape the bottom and sides of the melting pot to remove every last bit of these impurities before pouring into a mold. The final product should be a bright silver color.

The Casting Process

It is important to follow the manufacturer's instructions completely when using a bullet mold. Some will recommend heating the mold; some will recommend using a release agent, beforehand.

Whether the caster is filling the mold from a bottom spout or using the ladle, the molten lead needs to be poured directly into the hole on the top of the mold's sprue plate until there is a slight overflow (which is called sprue and how the plate gets its name). This will allow the mold cavity to fill properly as the lead cools.

The bullet will take its shape in about five to seven seconds. The caster can then rotate the sprue plate by tapping on it with a wooden dowel or a rubber or wood mallet. The sprue plate should cut the excess lead from the top and the open mold should release the bullet. The bullet may need to be tapped free of the mold by using the mallet again.

Your first bullets may have a crackled or wrinkled appearance due to the mold being too cool. Eventually the mold will achieve the proper temperature and the bullets will look fine. If they take on a frosted appearance it means the mold is getting too hot.

These newly formed bullets should be dropped into a towel, wooden box or in some instances, a pan of water to quench the bullets. The excess lead sprues can be added to the melting pot along with any flawed bullets and melted again to make new ones.

The bullets should be allowed to cool down and set for at least 24 hours before hand loading. In most cases the bullets will be ready to go at this point. If the bullets prove to be inaccurate, they may need to be resized to fit the firearm's bore. There are specialized motorized tools that can be bought for this purpose for under $1000 or the bullet caster can purchase a bullet sizing die of the appropriate diameter and mount it in a single stage reloading press in order to process several batches of properly sized bullets.

If you wish to size and lubricate the bullets, there is a specialized tool for this or the bullets may be lubricated individually. Spray lubricants can be applied or the caster may want to take another step and apply a coating.

Swaging Bullets

Bullet swaging is an alternative method of producing bullets at the individual level. It is mostly used by major ammunition manufacturers with expensive machinery and dedicated factories. Swaging utilizes pressure to form a bullet. As opposed to casting, no heat is needed and there is no requirement to melt the lead. Of course this negates the ability to use recycled materials such as dive weights, wheel weights, fishing lures or previously fired bullets, but it is the way to go if the hand loader wants to produce jacketed ammunition or specialized bullets such as a hollow based wad cutter. For making effective use of pre-existing materials, previously fired brass rim fire cases can be recycled and used as jacket material.

The pressure to swage a bullet is applied by means of either a hydraulic or hand-powered press. The press holds a die and a set of internal and external punches. The two punches apply force against the material from both ends of the die until it flows and takes on the actual shape of the die. When manufacturing a jacketed bullet, the lead core or wire is forced into the jacket material in the same manner.

Swaging can be performed in a home workshop using machinery made by companies such as Corbin. Most of the presses used for reloading can be used in the swaging process to swage the bullets, form bullet jackets from copper strip or tubing and make the lead wire, itself. Corbin offers dedicated swaging presses that can be easily converted to single stage reloading presses as well.

The initial set-up of a swaging operation is more costly than a basic casting venture, but can be more versatile, particularly if the end user has a greater need for jacketed ammunition for use in semiautomatic rifles and handguns. There is a reduced risk of exposure to toxic substances and the operation can be conducted "under the radar" with no one being the wiser to a manufacturing facility as they would with the smell of melting lead ingots. The end-user does not have to be concerned with fluctuations in the molding and casting process due to temperature, either.

After the initial cost of setting up the machinery, the cost of bullet production is essentially the same cost as the raw materials and the end result is usually a more accurate bullet as opposed to a cast bullet.

Machining Bullets

In some instances, bullets can be machined. Although it is not an ideal situation, it can be a method of last resort. We know several shooters of 338 Lapua Magnum and 50 BMG who have found it cheaper to turn out bullets for these rifles on a lathe or a screw machine. Some use bronze or copper and one uses steel in his 50 BMG rifle. The problem with steel is that it quickly erodes the bore of the rifle; however the shooter in question maintains that he spends so little on reloading components that he finds it cheaper to replace the barrel after it is shot out.

The Final Word on Lead Bullets

Lead is a toxic substance that can cause health problems and birth defects. It is advisable to wear gloves whenever possible while handling it and strongly advised for reloaders to wash their hands with cold soapy water after handling it and before eating drinking or enjoying tobacco products.

Powder

Gunpowder is an invention that traces its history to centuries before firearms development, much like the parachute was invented before the concept of airplanes. There are numerous types of powder available to the reloader and each one has its own properties.

It would be exhaustive and a waste of the reader's time to list every brand of propellant that is available. So we will go over the basics.

Black Powder

For over 600 years, black powder was the only small arms propellant available. In those six centuries it was noted for being hydroscopic and dangerous for the shooter to use. Black powder or its equivalent can be purchased today and is mostly used in muzzle loading firearms and certain black powder cartridges from the 19th century.

Black powder can be made from charcoal, sulfur and saltpeter. As it is an explosive and potentially dangerous, its manufacture is beyond the scope of this chapter

Smokeless Powder

After the discovery that burn rates of powder could be controlled by changing the granule size of the powder, Viellie and Nobel introduced smokeless powder to the world. This new powder did not have the corrosive or hydroscopic properties of black powder and most importantly it did not leave clouds of white smoke in its wake when a round was fired.

Because of the higher pressure involved with smokeless powder, it should only be fired in modern firearms made after 1898 and never fired in firearms marked "For Black Powder Only".

Primers

Of all the components that make up a round of ammunition, primers tend to be the most dangerous to handle or attempt to make.

Primer Size

There are three sizes of primers: shotgun, small and large.

Small and large size primers each come in three different degrees: rifle, pistol and Magnum. The size of the primer depends on the case.

Most center fire pistol ammunition uses the small pistol primer with the exception of 10mm, 45 ACP, 44 Special, 41 Magnum, 44 Magnum, 45 Colt, 45 ACP, 50 Action Express, 500 Smith & Wesson, 454 Casul and Wildcat cartridges based on these case designs.

Small Magnum primers are used by 357 Magnum and the large Magnum primers are intended for 41, magnum, 44 Magnum, 454 Casul, 50 Action Express and 500 Smith & Wesson when used in conjunction with a slow burning

powder that takes up almost all of the capacity of the case to guarantee proper ignition.

Shooters looking to save money should know that using a case loaded with a small amount of a fast burning powder does not require the more expensive Magnum primer.

Magnum primers should be used when the temperature is below 0 degrees and is safe to use with any ball powder. It may not be particularly advantageous to use with a fast burning powder and despite their expense, they may be the only primer that is available to the reloader.

The bottom line is that they are completely safe to use in non-Magnum rounds despite their ominous sounding name.

Shotgun primers are used for reloading shotgun shells and are used in lieu of percussion caps in certain inline modern muzzle loading rifles. They cannot be used to reload pistol or rifle ammunition.

HOW OUR ANCESTORS MADE HERBAL POULTICE
TO HEAL THEIR WOUNDS

"All that man needs for health and healing has been provided by God in nature, the challenge of science is to find it." - Philippus Theophrastrus (1493-1541)

When I was a little girl and I had fallen down and hurt my knee (it's always your knee you hurt when you're a child) my mother would put a poultice made of bread, warmed in milk onto the cut. It instantly soothed the knee. She'd leave it on, covered by a piece of material wrapped around it to hold it in place and keep the heat in. When I took it off, hours later, my knee definitely felt much better.

The art of the poultice is part of the long history of folk medicine that human beings have used since we came to be. Folk medicine is a way of healing, using things like plants and herbs as well as certain practices like blood-letting to fix an ailment.

The methods, recipes and techniques are usually passed down through generations. You may think that the ingredients in a poultice wouldn't really have any effect, but if you explore the ingredients and compare them to modern medicines you may be surprised at the similarities. For example, a poultice I mention in the section on recipes below contains opium. A medicine, available over the counter in a number of countries called 'kaolin and morphine' is used for a similar ailment and uses morphine (a related drug to opium and also derived from poppy seeds). Poultices may be seen to be 'folk medicine' but they work in similar ways to modern medicine and from my own experience, for certain ailments, they do just as good a job.

What is a Poultice?

A poultice is a topical application, often heated, and used to treat wounds and sores. The base of a poultice is often bread – like the ones my mother and grandmother would use. But bran and other similar cereals can also be used as the base. The Native Americans would use mashed pumpkin instead of bread.

The poultice ingredients would be heated, often in milk and the warm mash would be wrapped around the affected area using some sort of cloth – my grandmother would use rough linen or gauze.

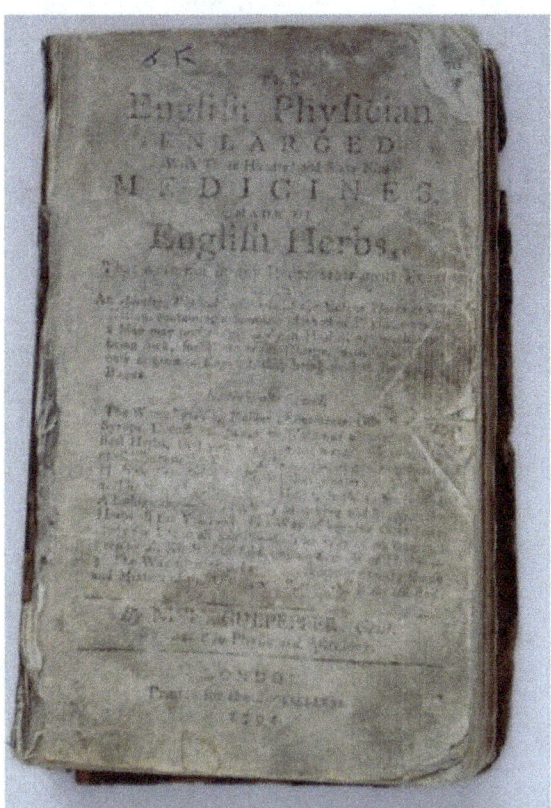

I have a book; it is dated 1794 and called "Medicine Made of English Herbs". The famous English herbalist, Culpepper, wrote it. The book has a small chapter on poultices and I will quote you a little piece from that, which explains what a poultice is and what it is used for (note that the book is written in old English using F instead of S, so I will translate into our more modern spelling):

"Poultices are those kind of things which the Latins call Cataplasmata, and our learned fellows, that if you can read English, that's all, call them Cataplasms, because it is a crabbed word few understand; it is indeed a very fine kind of medicine to ripen sores"

Original text:

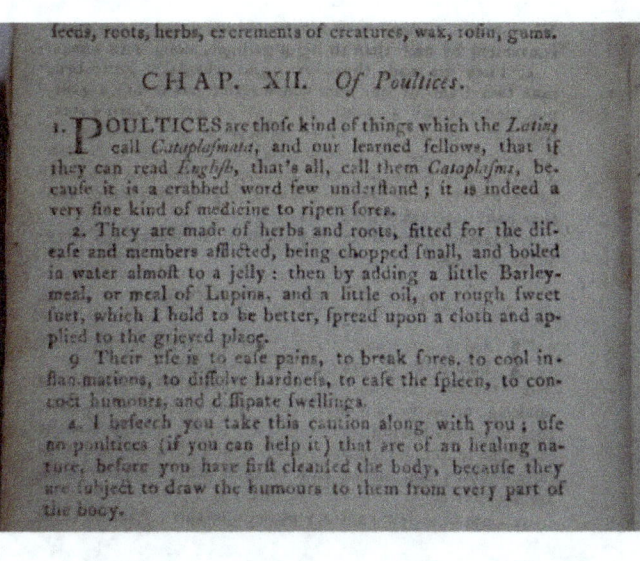

The poultice used by my grandmother and my mother was the same as that used by the likes of Culpepper in the latter half of the 18th century. It had stood the test of several centuries because it was effective. The recipes for poultice or Cataplasms are sometimes simple, sometimes complex. Their active ingredients vary, depending on the needs, but heat when used, plays a different role and acts as an activator for the ingredients and helps with blood flow and the movement of essential cells like antibodies and blood cells into the area. This is a way of speeding up the natural process of healing. Your body, when wounded produces heat as a way of encouraging the movement of cells; a poultice works in the same way. The recipes may be old, but the theory behind them is modern.

A Few Poultice Recipes

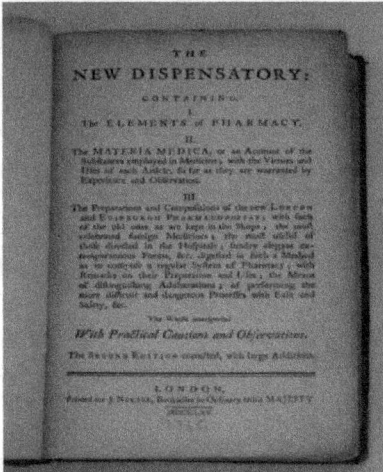

Another old recipe book, written in 1795 for pharmacists and entitled, "New Dispensatory" has a chapter on 'Cataplasms' with some interesting recipes. I've listed a few here to give you some ideas, but I'm sure you could modify these and perhaps come up with some of your own too.

Cataplasma Aromaticum

Aromatic cataplasm

- Long birthwort root[7];
- Bay berries[8], each four ounces;
- Jamaican pepper;
- Myrrh, each two ounces;
- Honey, thrice the weight of the powders.

Mix and make them into a cataplasm; which supplies the place of theriaca[9] for external purposes.

Soothing Poultice:

Cataplasma Emolliens - Emollient cataplasm

Take of

- Crumb of bread; eight ounces;
- White soap[10]; one ounce;
- Cow's milk, fresh, a sufficient quantity.
-

---

[7] Birthwort root has a lot of positive health benefits as it is anti-inflammatory, but it mustn't be consumed orally as it can be poisonous. Birthwort poultices were used by the native Americans to treat snakebites

For Stomach Aches:

Cataplasma Stomachicum - Stomachic cataplasm

Take of

- ❖ The aromatic cataplasm; one ounce;
- ❖ Expressed oil of mace; two drams;
- ❖ Anodyne balsam[11], as much as is sufficient to reduce them into a proper consistence

A Mustard Poultice

... which can be used for sore muscles, aches and pains and even chest congestion:

Sinapismus - A sinapism. Take of

- Mustard seed, in powder
- Crumb of bread, each equal parts;
- Strong vinegar, as much as is sufficient.

Mix and make them into a cataplasm; to which is sometimes added a little bruised garlic.

(As an aside, I was prescribed a very similar concoction to this by a physiotherapist I was seeing for back pain recently, it worked wonders)

A Native American Recipe to Treat an Abscess:

There is a tradition amongst Native Americans that was then inherited by the settlers of using a poultice. As mentioned earlier the poultice would often be made using a base of mashed pumpkin. But other base ingredients such

---

[8] Bay berries are from the bay tree and must not be consumed orally

[9] The word theriaca simply refers to the creation of a concoction

[10] White soap can be obtained as the soft froth you get when olive oil based soap is steeped in water for a long time

[11] Anodyne balsam, now this may be tricky to get as it does contain opium!

as cornmeal would also be used. Here is a recipe for a Native American Poultice used for abscesses:

Take:

- ❖ Cornbread, flaxseed or mashed pumpkin
- ❖ Ninebark decoction (steep the ninebark for several hours then decant the liquid)

Warm the decoction with the mash and place on the abscess.

A Word of Warning from The Past

A final word from the great herbalist Culpepper who says on the matter of Poultices in his 1794 book that:

"I beseech you take this caution along with you; use no poultices (if you can help it) that are of a healing nature, before you have first cleansed the body, because they are subject to draw the humours to them from every part of the body".

A warning to heed; the power of the poultice is great and should be used knowing that to be true. Use them wisely.

WHAT OUR ANCESTORS WERE FORAGING FOR OR HOW TO WILDCRAFT YOUR TABLE

"And God said, Behold, I have given you every herb bearing seed, which is upon the face of all the earth, and every tree, in the which is the fruit of a tree yielding seed; to you it shall be for meat." - Holy Bible: King James Version

Wildcrafting is simply collecting wild edibles from your environment. This is something everyone knew about at one point in human history. Food grows everywhere humans have settled. If you ever find yourself in a survival situation for an extended period of time, you'll be downright grateful for a salad of fresh greens or a tuber or two to supplement your rations. In fact, when you learn to identify the wild edibles in your region, you'll gain so many options to add variety to your food stores that you won't ever have to worry about burning out on the same 4 flavors of MRE's that you have had stored in your cellar since 1999.

The following list of herbs is far from comprehensive. All were chosen because they are found widespread across the United States and because they were most preferred by our grand-grandfathers. There are many wonderful plants that only grow in specific regions. Be sure to do a little research to discover what delicacy is growing near you, mayhaps in your own back yard. Still, the following plants should get you started and once you see how easy it is to wildcraft your table, you might find that you can't take a stroll in the woods any longer without bringing a harvest home for supper.

Arrowhead (Sagittaria Latifolia)

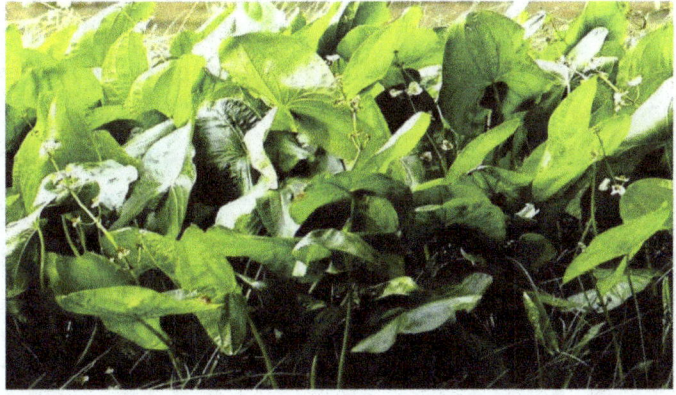

Perennial herb; Harvest all year. [12]

---

[8] "Sagittaria latifolia Willd", by: Udo Schmidt, (CC BY-SA 2.0)

Arrowheads are common. They grow in wet soil along creeks and rivers, in marshes and wetlands. They are easy to identify by their arrow shaped leaves. They grow in drainditches and soggy meadows too. This habitat is lucky because that wet soil gives up the plant easily with a little digging. The simplest way to accomplish this is to roll up your britches and wade in. Use your toes to loosen the roots. The tubers are what you're after and these float to the surface when they are dislodged. The tubers are edible raw but better cooked. They can replace potatoes in any recipe but ought to be peeled before eating.

Asparagus (Asparagus Officinalis)

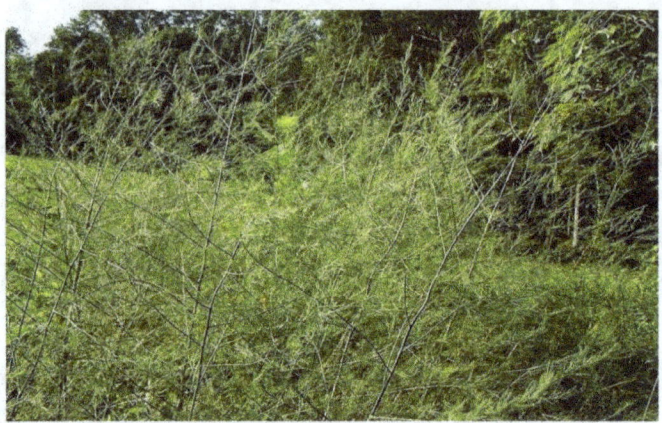

Perennial Herb; Harvest spring through summer.

Asparagus grows wild and is widespread throughout the continent. You will find it alongside roads, in ditches and anywhere else the soil has ever been disturbed. It prefers sandy, well-draining soil.

Harvest first in the spring, then all season long. Just be sure to give it enough time at the end to go to seed so there will be more next year. Don't eat older growth as it is mildly toxic. It's the young shoots you are after.

You can find asparagus by looking for the previous year's growth. You'll see dried, Christmas tree shaped stalks from the year before and if you look under and around them, you'll see the new shoots, especially early in the spring. Go ahead and cut all the stalks you see at ground level. They will grow back and you can continue to enjoy them all season.

Young, tender Asparagus is delicious raw. If you are on the go, it makes a delightful snack. If you are blessed enough to have some growing near your home/bunker or camp, keep an eye on it for new growth. You can chop it and toss it on a salad of wild greens for a treat.

_____

Asparagus is also great for soups. This is a great way to use them if you are lucky enough to find a good harvest. A cream of Asparagus soup is easy to make with just a few ingredients. Simply pour just enough water in the pot to cover the asparagus and boil it for 20 minutes or very soft. In another pot, place a pat of butter and a tablespoon of flour. When the flour is cooked through, pour the cooking water from the first pot, over the flour and whisk. Add enough milk to thin it to a nice consistency. Chop and mash the asparagus and stir it into the pot. Salt and pepper to taste.

Bulrush (Scirpus acutus, Scirpus validus)

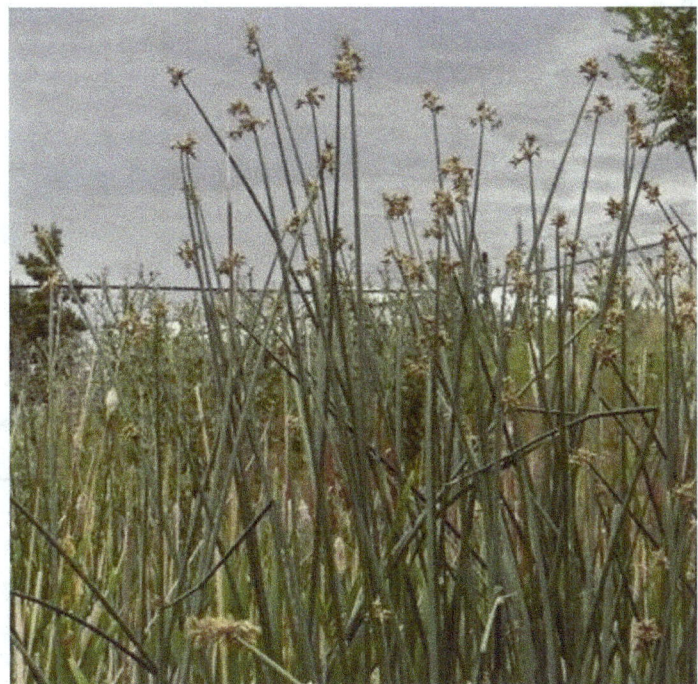

Perennial Herb; Harvest all year.

Every Plant in the Scirpus family is edible. So it doesn't really matter if you have an acutus or a validus on your table. The bulrush grows in the shallow water of marshlands or along the shore lines of any body of water. It starts at a tough underground rhizome that can be red or brown and grows straight up to a long, unbranched stem with one or no leaves and a flowering head.

Young shoots are edible raw. Older growth can still be eaten raw by peeling the stalks to reveal the tender core. These cores can be eaten like a salad, boiled or sauteed as any vegetable.

The roots of the bulrush are a nice treat. The young roots can be eaten like slender sweet potatoes or boil them for several hours to make a sugary sweet syrup. The older roots can be used as a starchy flour substitute by cutting and drying them, then grinding them. Remove fibers before storing the dry flour. The pollen and the ground seeds are excellent when added to dishes, including when using the roots as a flour substitute.

Cattails (Typha Latifolia, Typha angustifolia)

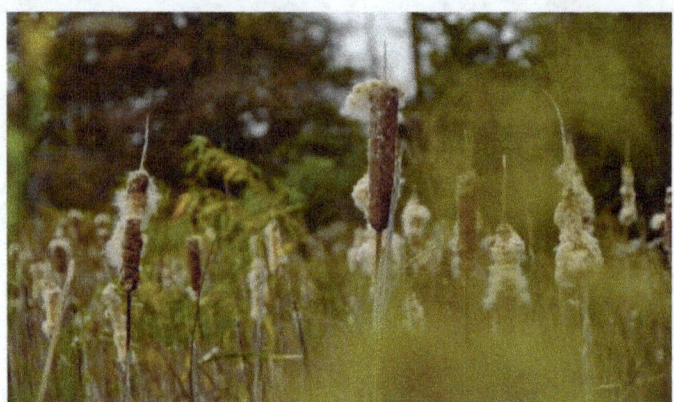

14Perennial Herb; Harvest all Year.

Cattails grow all over the continent. They are plentiful and easy to find. You'll most likely find Cattails near water. They like shallow water and marshlands the best. Identifying cattails should be easy. You will usually find old growth nearby and this will prevent you from mistaking them for their only poisonous look alike: the wild iris, which look remarkably similar along the roots and stems so be wary.

During the cold months, you can dig up roots. Roasted, these taste like a fibrous sweet potato or squash. It only takes a few minutes on an open fire to cook these through. Skin these roots and add them to your soup to thicken and add a satisfying starchiness.

In the early spring, you can dig at the roots to find dormant sprouts which are edible raw. As the season progresses, you can find these sprouts near the roots and leafy bases of the plant. Similarly, young stalks can also be eaten raw. Simply pull up the plant and peel back the leaves to reveal the young tender core. Both the sprouts and the core can be eaten alone or added to a salad.

The stalks and unripened blooms also make a great potherb which is cooked in a little water until tender. Less time for the stalks and a little more for the unripe blooms. Again, you'll want to peel the outer leaves first- a lot like an ear of corn, before cooking. In fact, when the blooms are tender, you can eat them just like you would corn on the cob or you can scrape the green buds off and use then in a casserole.

Once the pollen has ripened, collect the buds and remove it all. Carefully sift through the pollen to remove foreign materials and add it to your baking or sprinkle it over any dish for added nutrition.

Chickweed, Common

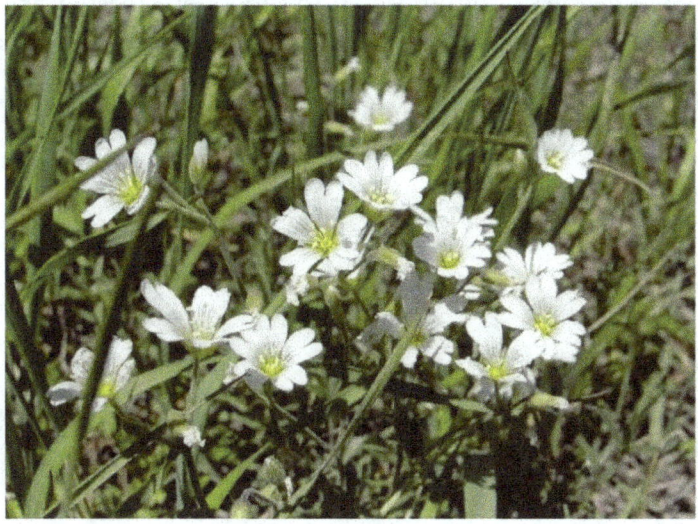

The easiest method of harvest is to pull up the whole plant and trim off the tender growth with scissors. You can get down on all fours and trim it the same way if you plan on harvesting the same plant later. Chickweed grows abundantly all across the continent so chances are that you'll know where several patches are growing at all times and there are no poisonous lookalikes so there is no reason not to harvest plenty. Look for it disturbed earth- yards, vacant lots, and road sides- but also where water grows, like near creeks and dark, moist spots in the woods.

The stems, leaves and flowers are edible, don't bother trying to separate them. Just chop it to bite size and enjoy as the base of a delightful salad. Or, if you'd prefer a cooked dish, you can boil them like you would any other greens, but only for a minute or two. I like to add them to a pot of other greens or my spring soups in the last few minutes. Another great way to enjoy them, especially if you have picky eaters, is to blanch them for a few minutes them blend them into pancake batter at a 1:1 ratio- one part chickweed, one part pancake batter. Cook them like regular pancakes and serve them warm, with a pat of butter and maple syrup. Then, pat yourself on the back for sneaking in some more healthy greens.

Chicory (Cirhorium Intybus)

Perennial herb; Harvest Spring, fall and winter.

Chicory was planted and harvested by pioneers as a coffee substitute. When the roots are roasted and ground, they taste like a slightly bitter black coffee. It now grows abundantly, everywhere. In the spring, before the plants get very big, you can take a knife and slice below the surface to gather the whole plant including the crown. These youngplants can be eaten raw in a salad as can the pale leaf crown all year. As they get older, the leaves become bitter so you may have to change the water if you collect them into the late spring. By summer, older growth is inedible. So stick with the new growth for salads.

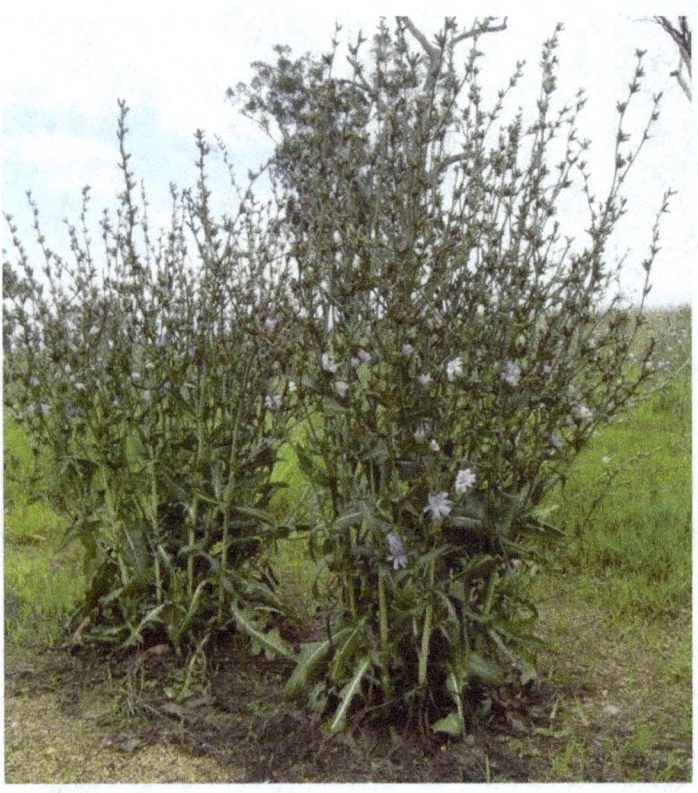

[16] Chicory plants yield tough roots that go deep into the soil. If you have soft soil, this isn't a problem but if you live in an area that's mostly clay, you should wait until after a good

_____

rain to try to harvest the roots. After roasting the roots, you'll need to grind them. Leave them coarse like coffee instead of grinding them to a powder.

Cleavers

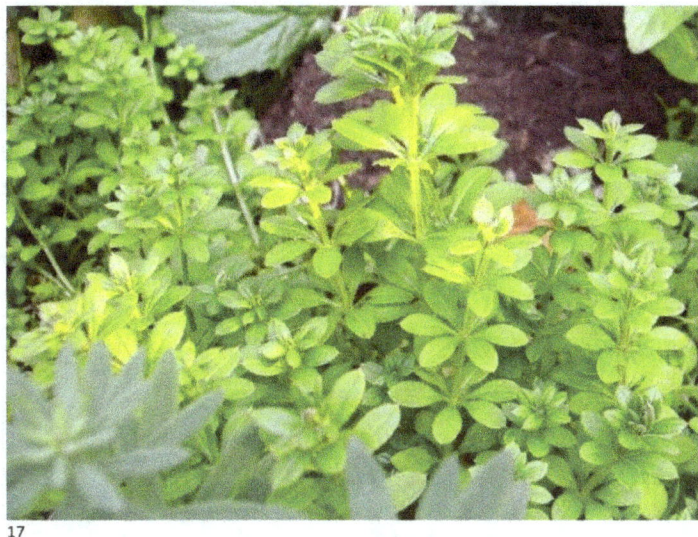
17

Annual herb; Harvest in the spring and summer.

Cleavers grow everywhere, especially in moist, rich soil. Harvest the young tender greens early in the season. You can steam these or boil them in a little water. These go nice in a cooked salad with asparagus and/ or potatoes (or arrowhead roots). Serve with a vinegar or mayonnaise based dressing. The fruits can be gathered in the summer.

_____

Roast and coarse-grind them and use them like coffee. They don't taste like coffee but they make a nice beverage, especially with a little honey.

Dandelion (Taraxacum Officionale)

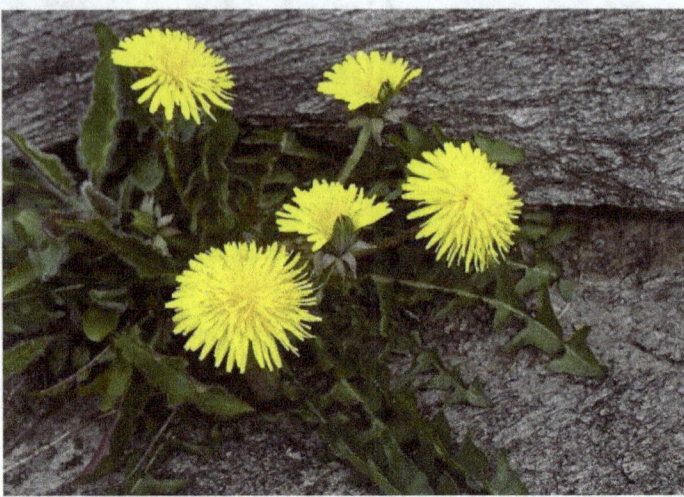

Annual or biennial herb; Harvest Spring fall and winter

The bane of green lawn enthusiasts, the dandelion might be the most well-known of the wild edibles.

The best time to use the greens are in the early spring while growth is still young and tender; these are great in a salad. Both young and older growth- to late spring, can be used as a potherb. You may need to change the water several times

_____

if it's really late in the season as dandelion greens get very bitter closer to summer.

Use the whole plant, including the flowers. In the fall, winter and very early spring, dig up the roots, including the leaf crown and new leaves (if any). Boil these in water for 20 minutes, changing water half way through. Dandelion flowers are a favorite to dip in batter and fry. If you are looking for a sweet treat, try these with honey or maple syrup. If you are looking for a savory snack, these are also excellent with garlic salt.

Henbit (Lamium Amplexicaule)

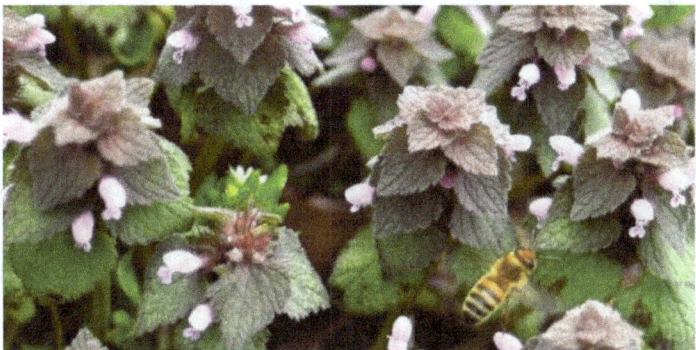

[19]Annual herb; Harvest in the spring.

Henbit is one of those that's hard to miss and easy to love. When we were small children we used to pick the dainty

_____

little purple flowers to eat in the play yard as a sweet treat. Now I pick the whole plant as a yummy green. Henbit is one of the early spring bloomers so it will also be one of the first herbs you identify each growing season. The shoots and young leaves make for a crisp and tender addition to a salad. The whole (above ground) plant can be used as a potherb.

Lady's Thumb (Polygonum persicaria)

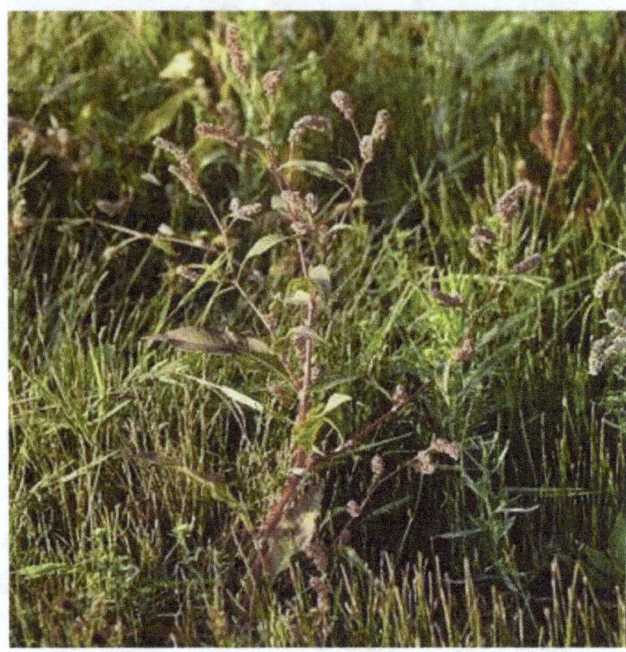

[20]Annual herb; Harvest in the spring through late fall.

_____

HOW OUR ANCESTORS NAVIGATED WITHOUT USING A GPS SYSTEM

"I may not have gone where I intended to go, but I think I have ended up where I needed to be." — Douglas Adams

Have you ever wondered how people used to find their way across the land or the seas without modern equipment? Not having a GPS might be doable but having no maps might be veering toward unbelievable. Still, we have no way of being sure that we will always have the comfort of either. After all, few people even own maps anymore, and our GPS system will be totally unreliable in case of an EMP. All that we'll know is what cities are north, south, east, or west.

Shadow Tip Method

This is based on the fact that the sun moves across the sky from east to west.

Materials:

- ❖ Stick
- ❖ Pebble

Procedure:

- ❖ Dig a small hole on the ground where you will stand the stick.
- ❖ Place the stick upright in the ground so that you can see its shadow. The narrower the tip is, the more accurate the reading will be.
- ❖ Make sure the shadow is cast on level and brush-free spot.
- ❖ Mark the tip of the shadow of the stick by scratching the ground or by using a pebble.
- ❖ Wait 10-15 minutes or just until the shadow tip moves a few centimeters.
- ❖ Mark the shadow tip's new position.
- ❖ Draw a straight line in the ground to connect the two marks to make your approximate east-west line.
- ❖ Label the first mark of the shadow as west and the second as east.
- ❖ Stand with the first mark, which is west on your left and the east mark on your right. The direction you are facing is north no matter where you are in the world.

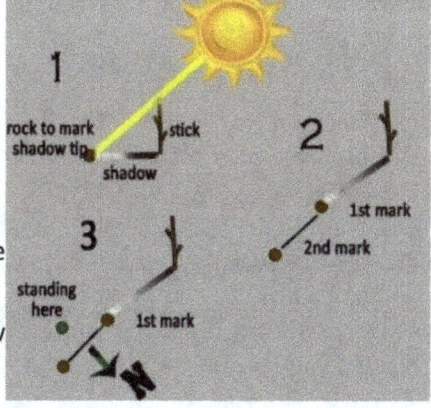

Watch Method

You can also tell the direction by using your watch Procedure:

- ❖ Make sure that the time is set accurately.
- ❖ Place it on a level surface or hold it horizontally in your hand.
- ❖ Position the hour hand of your watch toward the sun.
- ❖ Bisect or find the center point of the angle between the hour hand and the 12:00 mark.
- ❖ In your mind, draw the line based on the center point. This is the north-south line.
- ❖ If you're having trouble determining which way is north or south, remember that the sun rises in the east and sets in the west. It is due south at noon, east before noon, and west after noon.
- ❖ If your watch is set on daylight savings time, use the center point between the hour hand and the 1:00 mark to determine the north and south line.

Using the Stars

Because the North Star is known to stay fixed, is always visible in a clear night sky (from the northern hemisphere) and is always pointing north, our ancestors used it for thousands of years as a guiding star both on land and sea.

Finding the North Star was one of the basic skills all navigators and travelers knew and used on a regular basis; a skill that has been forgotten by the masses since the invention of the compass. But unlike the compass, the North Star always points to the TRUE NORTH. There is no magnetic declination to deal with.

The North Star, which is what we call it today, is actually named POLARIS (by astronomers), and surprisingly, it wasn't always The North Star and it won't always be:

"Thousands of years ago, when the pyramids were rising from the sands of ancient Egypt, the North Star was an inconspicuous star called Thuban in the constellation Draco the Dragon. Twelve thousand years from now, the blue- white star Vega in the constellation Lyra will be a much brighter North Star than our current Polaris. ... So when you're talking about stars "moving" or staying "fixed," remember ... they are all moving through the vastness of space. It's just the relatively short time of a human lifespan that prevents us from seeing this grand motion." [35]

One of the easiest ways to find Polaris is by using the group of stars known as the Big Dipper or the Little Dipper.

So you can go outside tonight (or now if it's already night) and try to find one of them first. The Big Dipper and the Little Dipper are actually the only groups of stars I know how to find. But I've known this since I was a little kid. It's very easy.

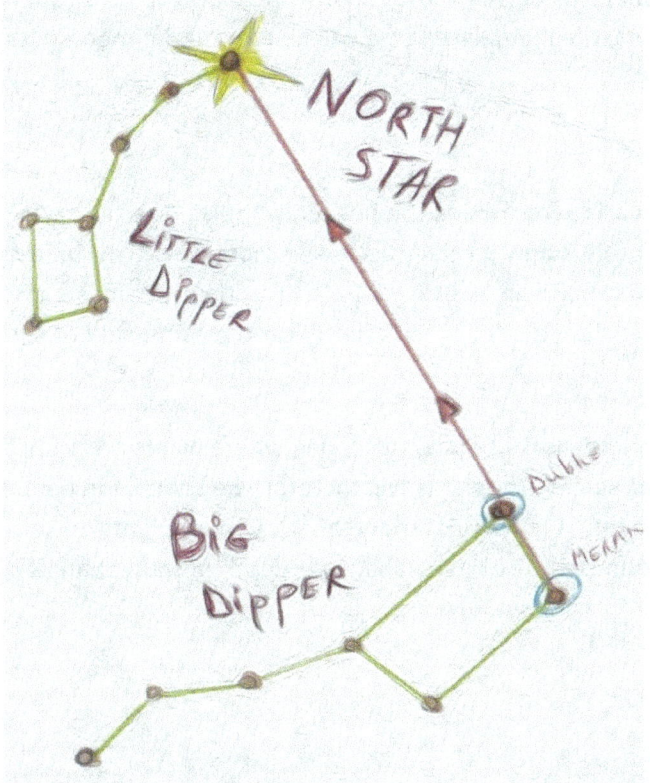

If you find the Big Dipper first, locate the two stars Dubhe and Merak in the outer part of the Big Dipper's bowl (see picture). Simply draw an imaginary line from Merak through Dubhe, and go about 5 times this distance to find Polaris.

If you find the Little Dipper first, Polaris is the last star in the handle of the Little Dipper.

After you find the star, stretch your arms sideways while facing it[36]:

- ❖ In front of you is True North.
- ❖ Behind you is South.
- ❖ Your right hand points due East.
- ❖ Your left hand points due West.

Letting the Sun Guide You

The important thing to remember when using the sun for navigation is that it will always rise in the general east and will set in the general west. Throughout the day the sun will make an arc to the south in the northern hemisphere and to the north in the southern hemisphere which will always be towards the equator. Deriving direction from these general facts, we can then say that in the morning, the sun will be in the general east, in the afternoon, it will always be in the general west.

If you determine that the sun is in the east, the north will be approximately a quarter turn counterclockwise. If the sun is in the west, then north will be a quarter of a turn clockwise. At around 12 noon, the sun will be due south in the northern hemisphere and due north in the southern hemisphere.

There are a few notes to consider. Seasons can change the path of the sun. During the summer, sunrise and sunset will be farther from the equator. In the winter, it will tend to be closer to the equator. And finally, during spring and fall, the sun will rise and set in the most accurate east and west.

---

[33] Added by the Editor

Letting the Moon Guide You at Night

When you're out during the night and the sun is nowhere to be seen, the moon can guide you to a rough east-west direction. If the moon rises before the sun sets, the illuminated side will be west. If the moon rises after midnight, the illuminated side will be east.

Moss and Other Vegetation

There's something we can learn from our grandparents aside from using the heavenly bodies. The old saying was that the moss grows on the north side of a tree but this is only partially accurate. Moss does grow on the north side of the tree but it also grows on the south and in every possible direction. To make our grandparents' saying more accurate, we should say that the equator is most likely on the same side of the tree where the moss growth is more lush and vigorous.

Another way to determine direction using vegetation and moisture is by observing where plants are damper. North- facing slopes receive less sun than south-facing slopes. The plants will therefore be cooler and damper on the north side. In the summer, north-facing slopes retain patches of snow. In the winter, plants on the south-facing slopes are the first to lose snow. The ground will also have a shallower depth of snow than its counterpart in the other direction.

Making a Compass

Materials:

- ❖ Metal sewing needle
- ❖ Cork or plastic bottle cap
- ❖ Bar magnet or ref magnet
- ❖ Sticky tack
- ❖ Shallow dish of water
- ❖ Sharp knife or scissors
- ❖ Towel (Optional)Procedure:

- ❖ Cut a circle approximately ¼ inch or 5-10mm thick from the end of a cork with scissors or a knife. You can also use an upturned plastic bottle cap.
- ❖ Place the product on one side.
- ❖ Magnetize the needle by rubbing it on the magnet from the tip to the bottom 50 times. If the magnet has its north pole labeled, then stroke the needle with this end. Remember to lift the magnet from the needle after each stroke to reduce the chance of de-magnetizing the needle as you return it back to the bottom.
- ❖ Stick the magnetized needle to the circle of cork with some tack. Alternatively, you can let the needle go through the cork.
- ❖ Float the cork in a dish of water.
- ❖ Keep the dish away from computers and other devices that contain magnets.
- ❖ Once it stops moving, the tip of the needle should be pointing due north and the tail pointing due south.

HOW OUR FOREFATHERS MADE KNIVES

- By M. Richard -

"A sharp knife is safer than a dull one." –
Unknown

The knife has been one of mankind's most essential tools since the first cave man found a stone that was brokento form a sharp edge and discovered how useful it was.
Since that time, countless designs of knives have been
made, in a constant effort to develop a better knife. Of course, there is no one perfect design, as knives are used for many different purposes.

Modern knives are made cookie-cutter fashion in factoriesaround the world. But in olden times, knives were each handcrafted works of art. While there were some factoriesthat made knives in the 1800s, these knives were thought to be inferior, useful only as trade goods with the Indians. Nobody who truly depended on their knife wanted a factory knife; they wanted one that was handmade by a skilled blacksmith or knife maker.

Today's factory produced knives are mostly ground from stainless steel, a material that didn't exist in the 1800s. While grinding has always been a necessary part of knife making, in times past knives weren't fully formed by grinding; but rather by forging.

Forging a Knife Blank

The beginning of any knife was making the blank out of highcarbon steel. High carbon steels were used, as they were harder and would hold a better edge. Steel making wasn't developed to today's highly scientific state and some knife makers would actually cast their own steel; however, the majority used the commercially available steels of the day.

Damascus steel blades were not common, except perhaps in Damascus. The basic difference between Damascus steeland other knife steel is that true Damascus steel uses morethan one type of steel, welded together so that the blade contains a combination of the characteristics of those steels. Hence, you could have a high carbon steel to give a good edge, welded to a more flexible steel so that the bladewouldn't break as easily.

Blacksmiths tended to reuse materials as well, especially inthe west, where materials shipments may not be as reliable. One favorite material for making knives was dull, used farrier's rasps (horse shoeing rasps). Most blacksmithshad a regular supply of these, made dull by shoeing the community's horses.

Farrier's rasps are still a popular blank for making knives today, as they are made of a very high carbon steel, which will make for a good knife blade. They are also larger than other files and rasps, making it possible to make larger knives out of them.

Forging the Blade

The knife maker would not cut the blade's shape out of the steel, regardless of whether he was starting with a fresh piece of steel or with a rasp; rather, the blank was heated in the blacksmith's forge and then shaped with hammer and anvil.

The point of a knife was formed by hammering the steel blank on the edges to narrow it down. This would cause the blank to thicken, so the hammering of the edges had to be combined with hammering the sides of the blank, thinning it back down. This process of stretching the metal while

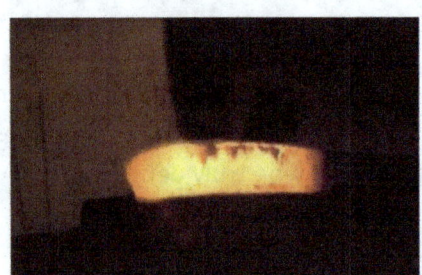

forming it is called "drawing" the metal. It is the blacksmith's standard method of changing the shape, thickness and width of a piece of steel.

Once the overall shape of the blade was established, the blacksmith would then move to tapering the blade. Once again, this was accomplished by drawing the metal, thinning it out. A lot of skill was needed to keep the blade's taper consistent during this process. Even so, most knives didn't have as clean a line down the side, where the flat meets the taper, simply because of the difference in manufacturing technique.

Final tapering of the blade was left for grinding. At this point, all the blacksmith was trying to do was to make the knife blank. The edge was usually left about 3/32" to 1/8" thick. A lot of grinding would be necessary to make it into a finished knife.

Forging the Tang

With the blade formed, the blacksmith would turn to shaping the tang for the handle. All knives made during this time period were full-tang knives. The idea of partial tang is an invention of industrialization, as a means of reducing costs. It was important to shape the blade first, as the handle would be made to balance the blade. Any extra material would be cut off the handle end, rather than the blade end.

Most knives had fairly simple handles, compared to today's knives. The idea of relieving the handle to create finger grips is relatively new in knife making history. Old knives had handles which were most often straight with a rounded end. Some might have handles which bowed out in the center or which had a wider butt to help maintain the grip.

As the knife blade had been drawn in forging, it would probably be wider than the unforged blank of the handle. However, for a very wide knife, the blacksmith might reduce the depth of the blade in essentially the same way that the point of the knife was formed, alternating hammering the edges and sides to draw out the steel to the desired shape. For fighting knives or sheath knives (which might also end up being used for fighting), the tang of the handle was forged to leave a step between the blade and handle, for a hilt to butt up against.

Finally, once the blade and handle are fully formed, the end of the handle is cut off to the right length for the knife's design and the end rounded.

Grinding the Blade

At this point, the knife maker just has a knife blank. The blade and tang are formed, but the blade is not sharp. The next stage in the process is grinding of the blade. In the 1800s, this was done on a foot powered grinding wheel, in the Middle Ages, they had to grind the blade on a rock to put an edge on it. Considering that the edge was roughly 1/8" in thick at the start of grinding, the process of grinding was a long one, which required a lot of patience.

The first step of grinding the blade is always to smooth out any inconsistencies in the blank's profile, both for the blade and the tang. The hammering of the blade can produce some slight waviness in the edge, which is eliminated by grinding. The final point of the blade is also formed at this point, as there are limits to what can be done on the anvil.

With the profile cleaned up, the knife maker moves on to grinding the taper of the blade. Knife makers did their grinding freehand, with the blade pointed up, just as experienced knife makers do so today. Considering that the average taper angle of a blade is somewhere between 7 and 15 degrees, maintaining that angle freehand is challenging, to say the least. Some knife makers used a block cut at an angle to ensure consistency, but this was a technique more for beginners, not experienced knife makers.

Grinding of the blade is accomplished by long strokes, the full length of the blade, rather than working on only one part of the blade. The long strokes across the grinding wheel help to keep the blade shape and edge consistent. Every few strokes the blade is flipped, allowing the other side to be ground. In this manner, the blade is kept even, so that the edge goes right down the center of the blade.

The knife is not fully sharpened in this stage, but the blade is ground to a fine edge. The actual cutting edge of a knife is usually 20 to 30 degrees, even though the blade makes a much sharper angle. Final sharpening is done by hand on a whetstone, as the very last step.

Hardening the Blade

The finished blade needs to be hardened and tempered to make it usable. The repeated heating and cooling of the metal during forging causes the metal to be annealed. This makes it easier to work and to bend, but is not good for a blade that must be kept sharp.

Before tempering, rivet holes are drilled in the tang. Most knives had two rivets in the handle, but it is possible to find examples with more. The rivets will hold the sides of the handle to the tang. For knife makers who did not have the capability of drilling holes (not all blacksmiths did), the holes could be made with a punch.

The process of hardening the blade consists of heating it and then quenching it in oil. This works better when the oil is hot, which is easily accomplished by heating an additional piece of steel in the forge and then running it through the oil bath to warm it.

A horizontal oil bath works better for hardening knife blades than a vertical one. What I mean by that is a bath that allows the knife to be placed in it horizontally, rather than vertically. Putting the knife in vertically, as if you were stabbing the oil can cause uneven cooling, which can warp the blade.

The blade is heated in the forge until it reaches a temperature where a magnet will no longer stick to it. Experienced knife makers can tell when it reaches this temperature visually, but the magnet is a good check for the temperature of the blade.

It is not uncommon to have the blade sitting in the fire in such a way that the cutting edge of the blade is in the coals, where it is getting the maximum heat, while the back of the

blade and the tang are not in the coals. This allows these parts of the blade to remain softer, so that the knife isn't brittle.

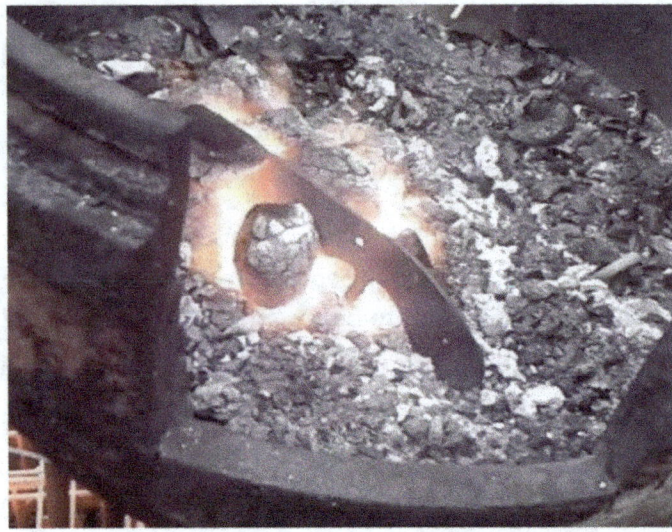

Properly heated, the knife blade will be glowing bright red, although the back and tang will not be. The blade is put into the oil bath slowly and evenly, edge first. The whole blade must enter the oil bath, but the most important part is the blade edge. The oil typically catches fire, so it is necessary to have a means of putting out that fire.

When the blade is removed from the fire it will have a scale all over it. This is easily cleaned up with a file. It is also brittle, so it needs to be tempered to make it less brittle. This requires a second heating, but to a much lower temperature. The metal was heated to about 1500 degrees and oil quenched to harden it, now it is heated to about 400 degrees for about two hours and allowed to air cool to temper it. The actual temperature used will depend on the type of steel used for the knife.

Making the Handle

Many different materials have been used through the centuries for knife handles. The simplest handle is created by wrapping the tang with leather, but wood is most common. Handles can also be made of antler, bone, stone and even the preserved feet of animals.

If the knife is going to have a hilt, the knife maker would cut it out of thick sheet metal, usually brass (1/8" to 1/4" thick). As a soft metal, brass works well for a knife hilt, as the opponent's blade may stick in it, when blocking, giving the knife wielder an opportunity to try and jerk the knife out of their opponent's hand.

Wood handles are made by rough-cutting the two sides, usually out of the same thin piece of wood. The knife tang is used as a pattern for cutting out the handle pieces and drilling the holes. Once rough shaped, they are attached to the handle with rivets (usually brass). Final shaping of the handle is made back on the grinder, shaping the handle to fit comfortably in the hand.

The final step to making any knife is to put an edge on it with a whetstone. Knife makers look for an ideal of an edge that can cut paper by being pushed through the edge of the paper, without any lateral movement. That's a really sharp blade.

To Make Your Own Knife

Most of us don't have a blacksmith's shop in our backyards, or even know how to work in one, if we did have it. So, we are limited in our ability to make knives. However, if you have a grinder or stationary belt sander, you can still make knives by grinding the blades. A belt sander actually works better and is the tool of choice for most modern knife makers.

While people who make knives regularly use some rather sophisticated belt sanders, you don't need a high dollar belt sander to make a knife. I have a 1" by 30" belt sander, which I bought at Harbor Freight. This is probably the cheapest belt sander on the market, yet I have been able to make knives successfully on it. The narrow belt actually works better than a wide belt would, more closely resembling the two inch wide belts used by the pros.

To start, use an old file for your steel. The knife shown below was made out of an old flat file I had sitting around. The first step is to draw out the shape of the blade on the knife. In this case, I'm making a small drop-point knife. The finished blade will be 3/4" wide and about 4" long.

This profile is then made on a grinder, removing all the material outside the drawn lines. Be careful to grind so that the edges are 90 degrees to the face of the blade. You will need to wear insulated leather gloves (such as welding gloves) or hold the knife blank with pliers to keep from burning your fingers on the hot metal.

Once the profile is shaped to your satisfaction, it's time to move on to putting the taper on the blade. This is most easily accomplished on the belt sander, using a block to hold the knife blank and maintain the angle. In the photo below, I've attached the knife to the block with double- sided masking tape. The taper on the block is five degrees,cut on my table saw.

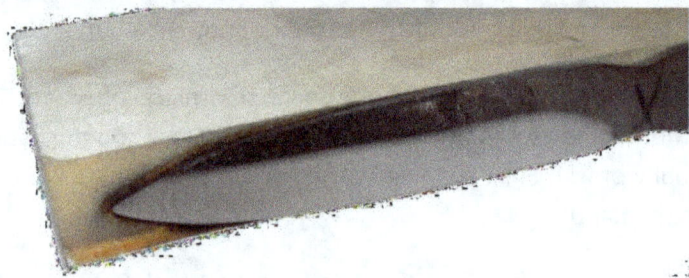

As you can see from the photo, it is fairly easy to maintain a clean line on the blade, if you use long strokes across the belt, while grinding. I took this blade down to a thickness of about 1/32" at the edge, before abandoning the belt sanderand finishing the edge on a whetstone.

If you can keep the blade cool while grinding, you may not have to reharden and temper it. Dipping it in cool water between grinding strokes can help with this. However, if your blade heats up to red even once, it will have lost its temper. This is, of course, more likely to happen at the point, rather than anywhere else. A clear indication that the blade has been overheated will be that the metal has turned blue.

If you have to harden your blade, you can accomplish the same sort of hardening with a small plumber's torch and Map Gas. Don't try it with propane, as it won't get hot enough to turn the steel red.

For the rest of the project, you can do things essentially the same way that they did it in olden times. Sharpening a knife on a whetstone hasn't changed much, nor have the methods for making a handle. You may decide to make a more complex handle shape than they did back then, but since you're grinding it, that won't be much of an issue.

Don't forget to make yourself a nice sheath to show off yournew knife. A sheath not only allows you to carry yourhomemade knife with you, but also protects the knife frominadvertent damage.

GOOD OLD FASHION COOKING ON AN OPEN FLAM

"One of the very nicest things about life is the way we must regularly stop whatever it is we are doing and devote our attention to eating." - Luciano Pavarotti

When planning for an uncertain future, the first thing you may want to do is build up your supply of food, but that act has little meaning if you have no way to cook it. Some serious preppers have already figured that problem out with alternative power sources and generators to run their electric ovens. The rest of us will have to make do with good old fashioned cooking on an open fire.

Home makers of the 18th and 19th century could turn out culinary masterpieces that were not only hardy, but so good the recipes have been copied, tweaked and handed down, generation after generation, until they reached the modern era of convenience foods and microwaves. Now, when you want a pie all you have to do is pop down to the grocery and pick one up. Something was lost when we gave up the old ways of cooking. Let's face it, food tastes better when it's lovingly created and carefully tended.

If you want to not only survive disaster, but to live and flourish, you'll want to learn to cook over an open flame like the pioneers did. With the right tools, heaps of patience, and just a little bit of practice, you'll be creating fire roasted feasts like you've been doing it your whole life.

Cast Iron Cooking

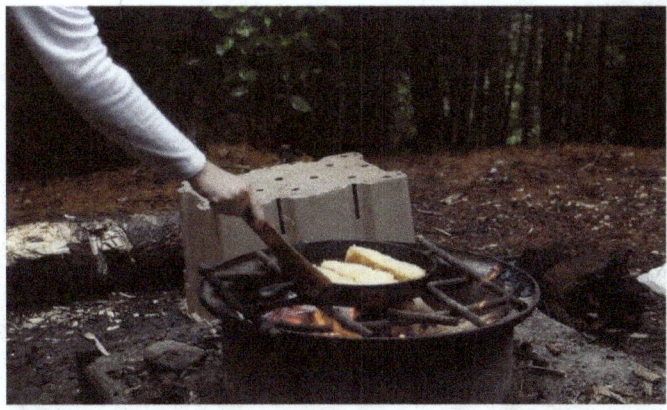

_____

Arguably the most important investment you can make to your well prepared survival kitchen is a good set of cast iron cookery. Some people will tell you that aluminum is better. The thought process there is that it is light and easy to carry. Many more think steel is the way to go. However, for durable, long lasting cookware that will only get better the more you use it, nothing compares to cast iron. Cast iron can stand up to the heat of open fire cooking and it is easy to maintain. Good cast iron is not cheap, but it's worth it to spend a little extra to get the good stuff. Otherwise you may wind up sitting there, years after the economy has crashed and the supermarkets are vacant, and you with a flimsy pot that has a gaping hole in it where your cast iron ought to be.

Care and Use

Okay, so now you know why you need cast iron. If you want your cast iron to be nonstick and easy to manage, there area couple of things you ought to know.

Seasoning your Cookery

If you buy your cast iron new, there will be instructions on how to season it included in the package. If you buy it used, chances are, it will already be seasoned. Either way, seasoning it is pretty simple and should be done regularly anyway. To season your cast iron, simply slather it in oil and stick it over hot coals to cook the oils in.

Never Use Dish Soap

Good cast iron is coated in oil. Dish soap breaks down oil; that's how it cleans. You want to avoid this at all costs. If you do accidentally use soap on your cast iron, rinse it immediately and rinse it well, and then be prepared to re- season it. If you are not careful, the soap will soak into the metal and taint your next meal. Instead of soap, use a good stiff brush or some steel wool. The settlers used wads of horsetail to scrub their pots and pans.

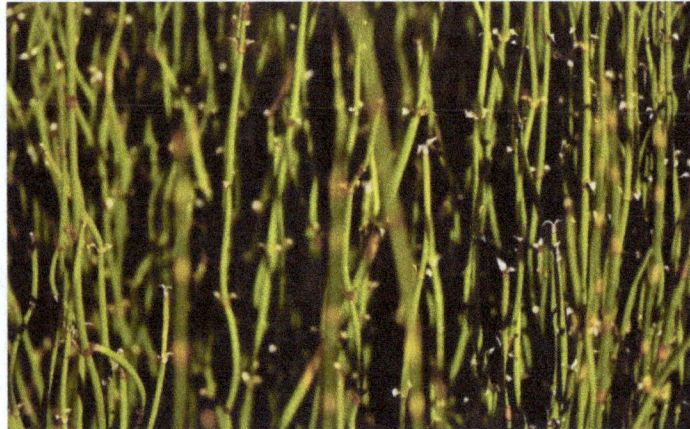

47

This highly fibrous plant works well and can be found abundantly in damp places. In this day of disinfectants and germ phobia, it may seem counter intuitive to NOT use soap, but trust me, the temperatures needed to cook your meals are hot enough to kill any potential germs and a well-

_____

seasoned cast iron surface should be easy enough to clean without soap.

Iron Rusts

Because iron does rust, never leave it soaking in water or water in it. Even if you think it is well coated with oil, it will rust. If you are not cooking with it, clean it, dry it, oil it down and put it away. Keep in the habit of taking care of your cast iron. If cared for properly, it will last for generations.

No Fire

Or at least, don't leave an empty pot in the fire. It's tempting, to just burn all the left-over food off, but cast iron can warp and even crack if left in a hot fire too long. For the same reasons, don't put cold water in a hot pan. Again, take care of your cookery and it will take care of you.

Companion Tools

If you are prepping a survival kitchen and you've got your cast iron, there are a few things you should think about packing with it. You'll need heavy pot holders, because good cast iron is all metal and those handles get HOT! If you ge cast iron cooking pot, you'll want a metal hook to remove it from the fire. They also make heavy hooks to remove t lid of your pot- sensibly called: lid lifters. Tongs, spoons, spatulas and other cooking utensils will also be necessary

Roasting Meats

This is always what I think of when I think of outdoor cooking. Roasting trophy catches over an open fire is the epitome of frontier cuisine. That said, if you've ever actually tried it, you'll know that it can be trickier than it looks. That's okay. Even roasting meat takes skill and know how. The know how you can get here. The skill will come with practice.

On a Spit

There is a wide variety of barbecue roasting spits available commercially or if you're handy, you can make a good one without too much trouble. In the wild, you can use sticks to construct a spit above your fire. Be sure to leave enough of the spit stick on the end, out of the direct heat to be able to easily turn it.

You should always use a thermometer when checking your roast. And in some cases, doneness is a matter of taste. You can gauge about how much time you need to wait by these approximate times:

- ❖ lamb: 30 minutes per pound
- ❖ beef: 20 minutes per pound
- ❖ pork: 45 minutes per pound
- ❖ chicken: 30 minutes per pound
- ❖ venison: 20 minutes per pound

Treat small game like lamb and expect 30 minutes per pound. Fish doesn't take as long, but because of the possibility of microscopic parasites, you want to be sure it's well done. When the skin peels off easily and the meat flakes, it should be ready to go.

On a String

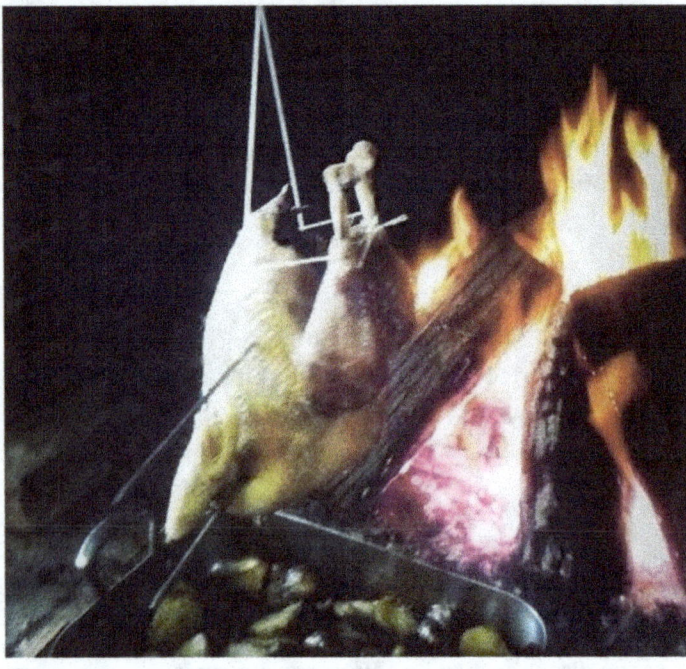
48

This is one of my favorite techniques for roasting smaller game, poultry and dinner sized roasts. If your cooking surface is your fireplace, then this is one cooking method

_____

you should familiarize yourself with immediately. It's easy and the meat comes out perfect with very little fuss.

Choose the right sized meats for this method. Don't choose heavy meats or you'll break your string. You don't want big roasts either, because the center will still be raw as the outside burns. Chicken is perfect. Small game and reasonable sized hunks of meat work too.

Once you've got your meat seasoned the way you like it, you will have to truss it up with some kitchen string. Either knot it well or go ahead and buy a set of trussing needles to attach the chicken to the string. You'll secure the legs and wings to the sides and hook it over the fire. If you have a wooden mantel, this is the perfect place to stick the hook. If you are outside, look for a good size branch or one of those iron hangers for hanging plants.

You'll want to place a drip pan under the meat to avoid any messes. As the string slowly unwinds, the chicken turns itself, making this a hassle free dinner. Every now and then, twist the string back up and while you're at it, baste the meat and string occasionally to keep them moist.

It takes around an hour and a half to roast a chicken, but you should use a thermometer to make sure.

Tips:

Let that fire burn for more than an hour before you start cooking; feeding it when needed so that there are plenty of hot coals and less open flame. You want the meat close enough to get the heat without the fire touching it.

No matter what you are roasting, you want to try to shape the meat so that it is as even and cylindrical as possible. That way, it will be evenly cooked.

Dutch Oven Cooking

Even if you forgo the cast iron skillet or soup pot, you should have a dutch oven. Not only can you bake in a dutch oven, but the body of the oven can be used for anything cooked in a pot and the lid can be turned upside down to be used like a frying pan. A dutch oven can do it all and then some. Cooking in a dutch oven may take some getting used to. Figuring out how to get and keep the right temperature takes time and patience, but if you take that time, and have the patience, you will be so happy with your dutch oven dinners that you won't even miss the modern convenience kitchens at all.

Choosing a dutch oven can be confusing. There are a lot of pots out there that call themselves dutch ovens, but they won't do for what you need. So, let's get some specifics down. Your dutch oven must be cast iron. It needs a tight fitting lid that is either concave or at least flattish with a lip. A dutch oven with feet is best, but one without will do too, and it only matters the size in the context of how many you are feeding and what you are making. I have a big family, so I have three: small, medium and large. With these, I can cook a feast.

Care of your dutch oven is the same as the care of the rest of your cast iron cookery. The same do's and don'ts apply.

The Right Temperature

Most guides and recipes that you will find online today talkabout dutch oven heat in terms of how many coals it takes:so many coals on top and so many on the bottom. Let's face it, most of us preppers are not going to keep a store ofcharcoal on hand just to cook in our dutch ovens. That's ridiculous. People used dutch ovens to cook with long before they could get standardized charcoal briquettes to barbecue with. The problem is that it's really hard to explain heat distribution in other terms, especially since different wood coals will hold heat differently.

[49]Think in terms of equal space. You'll usually want to use as many coals as it would take to completely fill in the spacebelow your oven. Distribute the coals according to the

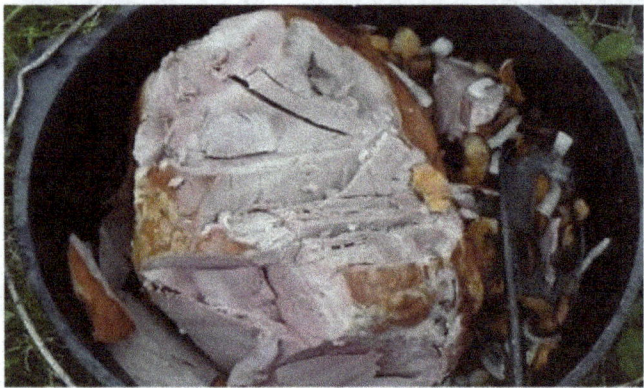

guidelines below. Adjust the amount as you see fit afteryou gain a little experience.

Roasting: Using the starting amount of coals, put half ontop and half on the bottom.

Baking: Put a quarter of your coals on the bottom and 3/4ths on the lid.

Simmering: Place 3/4ths of the coals on the bottom and aquarter on top.

Frying: Put all your coals on the bottom

***Always space your wood coals evenly apart for the bestresults.

Companion Tools

There are plenty of good accessories to go with your dutch oven. Depending on your cooking preferences, some of these will be more useful than others.

leather gloves- and heavy potholders to handle a hot oven

a lid lifter- a long metal hook used to remove the lid to yourdutch oven safely

a small shovel- used to move coals around

a trivet- when baking or steaming in your dutch oven, a trivet will keep your food off the hot sides

_____

a cake pan- placed on the trivet, you'll want a pan that is slightly smaller in diameter than your dutch oven.

Tongs - long handled tongs are an invaluable tool for cooking over a fire in any cookery

Other utensils- as you would always use, spoons, spatula, etc.

Recipes Past and Future

These recipes were chosen to be easy and without too many exotic ingredients (sans spices- stock up on those!). With that in mind, enjoy the fruits of your labors. Your larder is well stocked and your garden growing well. You deserve a feast.

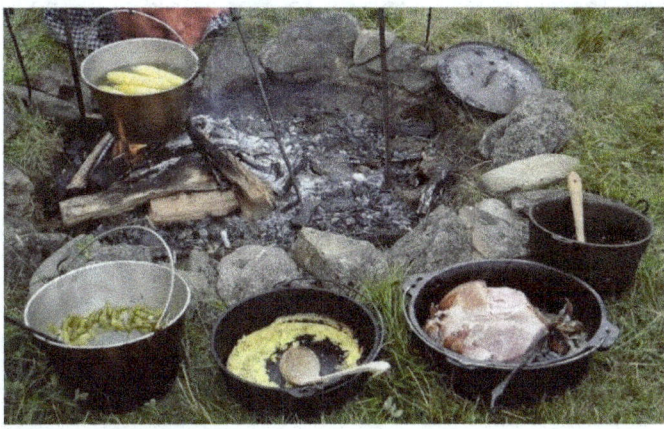

Colcannon

Colcannon is a traditional Irish dish that's more brilliant for its simplicity. Boil a head of cabbage and twice as many potatoes as the size of the cabbage until good and soft. Chop and mash them together and season with salt and pepper. Traditionally, colcannon was served with a healthy dollop of butter and cream.

Meat Pies

These are a beautiful way to use left-over meats, especially roasts, and stews.

Crust - Mix some flour with a little salt and some fat (butter, lard, whatever) until a stiff paste is formed. Use this to line the bottom of your pan and if you have enough, cover the top of the pie too.

Filler- Use whatever meats and vegetables you have on hand. Thicken some broth or drippings with some cooked flour, mix it all together and pour it over the crust.

You can cook this right in your dutch oven if you like, or in the cake pan if you want a smaller amount. Bake it for more than an hour, until everything inside is tender and the crust is crisp. Turn-overs are made with the same ingredients, but you make a big, flat crust and spoons some filling in the middle of one half. Fold the crust over and pinch it together, and then cook it on a frying pan turn-overs were a popular meal to send off with working men and will hold well for a day or so if prepared in advance.

Mock-mock turtle soup:

Original mock turtle soup called for a calf's head to be boiled down for 8 hours. In this recipe, we'll use whatevermeat we have on hand. Boil a pound or more of meat- withthe bones, if you have them, for at least 2 hours. The watershould be seasoned with bay, parsley, marjoram and basil (okay, use what you've got). After 2 hours, toss in enough root vegetables, such as potatoes, turnips and carrots, to feed your family. While this is cooking, take 6 hard-boiled egg yolks and mash them together with a little raw yolk andsome flour to make a dough. Roll a dozen marble sized balls and toss them into the pot with a cup or two of red wine when the vegetables are almost tender.

Wassail:

The Wassail bowl is a forgotten Christmas tradition. Even the old cookbooks refer to it as an old one. The spicy drink was ushered in with much ceremony, often decorated with wreathes and ribbons. It would be a beautiful tradition to bring back when we find ourselves in need of a little reminding about the good things in life.

Many old recipes can be found for wassail. Depending on the cook, it might have beer, cider or wine as the base. Thespices vary too. Feel free to adapt and change the followingrecipe to include whatever you have on hand and to satisfyyour own taste buds. This is as much of the tradition as drinking the wassail itself.

In a small pot, boil:
- 1 tsp. Cardamon
- 1 tsp. Clove
- 1 tsp. Nutmeg
- 1 tsp. Mace
- 1 tsp. Ginger
- 1 tsp. Cinnamon
- 1ts. Coriander
- in a cup of water.

After about 20 minutes, pour it into a gallon of wine/beer or cider. Add 3 to 4 cups of sugar. And put in on the fire.

While it is cooking, prepare the wassail bowl by cracking a dozen eggs into it and beating them well. Add a cup of thewarming wine to the eggs and beat it in. Repeat this step three more times.

Then, when the wine begins to boil, take it off the heat andpour it gradually into the bowl, taking care to go slow and stir continuously. You need to stir briskly to form the froth that makes wassail so pretty.

Once you have it poured and frothed, serve it immediately. Roasted apple or a couple cups of raisins were commonly tossed in the wassail. A pint of brandy was also often foundthere.

Apple Pie

Prepare a stiff paste for the crusts by mashing flour into fat (butter, lard, shortening). Line your well-oiled dutch oven with the paste, reserving enough for the top. Make sure the crust is as even as possible. Roll the rest out to make your top crust. You only want your pie to be an inch or twothick. Three max.

Peel, slice and core your apples. You can parboil or stew them in a little water but if they are very ripe, this is not necessary. Add cinnamon, sugar and butter to taste.

Dampen the top of the crust in your dutch oven, lay your top crust on top and pinch them together. Cut a slit on topto vent, put the lid on your oven and place it in the coals with a quarter of the coals on bottom and the rest on top. It takes 45 minutes to an hour to bake a pie this way.

***If you are using dried apples, reconstitute them and stew them for an hour or so before adding them to the pie.You should stew unripe apples as well.

Biscuits and gravy

Start this recipe with a well-oiled dutch oven. Preheat it keeping all of the coals on the bottom to get it nice and hot.While it's heating up, mix together in a bowl:

- ❖ 2 c. Flour
- ❖ 1 tsp. Salt
- ❖ 1 tbs. Sugar
- ❖ 4 tsp. Baking powder.
- ❖ Cut in 1/3 c. shortening
- ❖ Then add ¼ c. milk. Mix only until everything is wet.

Spoon drop the biscuits into the dutch oven, evenly spacedand put on the lid.

Now, remove ¾ of the coals from under the oven, taking care to even out the remaining coals. Put the ¾ coals you took out from under, on top. Bake for 8-10 minutes or untilgolden on top. Remove and cover with a towel to keep warm.

Put the coals back under the oven and add your meat. I likepork sausage, but grandma sometimes used pork chops or just plain lard when there were none. Cook thoroughly. If you are using just a fat to make this gravy, and maybe if youaren't, you'll want to season it with sage, thyme and onionas well as salt and pepper.

Add ¼ c. of flour to the pot and stir until well cooked, but not burnt. Then add 2 ½ c. milk and stir until thickened. Serve immediately by pouring over the biscuits on individual plates.

Easter Cake

Using this method, you can bake any and all of your favorite cake recipes in the dutch oven. This Easter Cake is an adaptation of a recipe found in the 1903 Boston Cooking- School Magazine. During times of crisis, there is little that says, "Everything is going to be okay." like a bit of cake. It seems cake just brightens the dreariest of days.

Preheat your dutch oven using half and half for the coals. Use a trivet in your oven. If you don't have a trivet, similarsized pebbles, marbles or beads work well too.

Sift together 1c. flour with 1 tsp. Baking powder. Set aside. In a separate bowl, beat 4 egg whites until stiff. In yet another bowl, beat ½ c. soft butter with ½ .c sugar. Add 1 tsp. Vanilla extract. Combine all ingredients and mix well.

You need a cake pan that is smaller than your dutch oven. A 9 inch cake pan and a 10 inch dutch oven are ideal. Pour your batter into a greased cake pan. Pour an inch of water into the bottom of your dutch oven and place the pan on the trivet. Leave the coals half and half for this recipe. It takes 45 minutes to 1 hour for the cake to be done.

Porridge

There is little more versatile than the porridge. It can be made using oats, rice, buckwheat or any other grain. It can even be made using peas. The porridge was a traditional mid-day meal for peasants in Europe and the settlers of early America. This recipe makes the best breakfast porridge ever.

In the evening, dig a small ditch near your fire pit and line it with hot coals. Combine in your dutch oven, 1 c. of rolled oats with 4 c. water and 2 c. milk. Add 1 c. applesauce and 1 cinnamon stick. Put your dutch oven in the pit and cover it with more hot coals. Then bury it with dirt. In the morning, uncover the dutch oven, being especially careful not to dislodge the lid. Dust off the dirt and ash before serving (no one wants ashy porridge).

Stew

Like the porridge, stew is a favorite of days gone by. A stew is rather easy to make. In the morning, toss whatever meats and vegetables you have on hand in a pot along with your favorite seasonings and cook it on a medium fire for most of the day. An hour before it is to be eaten, thicken it with cooked flour, cornstarch, arrow root, mashed beans or potatoes. Serve and enjoy. Stews go particularly well with bread.

Bread

Making in a dutch oven is easy! The trick is not to be too much of a bread snob. Use bread flour if you can get it. All-purpose works fine when you can't. Whole wheat works good too when you are using this method.

Start the day before you want to eat the loaf. Combine:

- ❖ 3 c. Flour
- ❖ 1 tsp. Yeast
- ❖ 1 tsp. Salt
- ❖ 1 ½ c. Water

In a large bowl, mix until everything is wet, but don't worry too much about the lumps. Set the bowl aside in a warm, safe spot and forget about it.

The next day, an hour before you want to bake, preheat your well-oiled dutch oven with half the coals on top and half on bottom. Meanwhile, turn your dough out onto a floured surface and gently (DO NOT KNEAD) shape it into a roughly dutch oven shape. You want it kind of evenly flat on top. If it rises too much, it will stick to your lid!

Move your coals back into baking position and bake for 45 minutes.

LEARNING FROM OUR ANCESTORS HOW TO PRESERVE WATER

"We never know the worth of water till the well is dry."

- Thomas Fuller 1732

There is an old Slovakian proverb that sounds something like this "Water is the world's first and foremostmedicine." It couldn't be more right.

The Law of Three states that survival is only possible for three weeks without food, three days without water, and three hours without warmth. This law illustrates the importance of water to humans. Even without any source of food for three weeks, a person cannot survive without water after three days. We all know that water is essentialto our daily lives, but in the event of a disaster that could potentially endanger everything that we need for survival,

it's necessary to know how to get safe and clean drinking water.

Before there were long-term settlements, our ancestors would often set up camp or stay in a place where there wasa nearby water source. This means that a whole tribe or group had to have the knowledge of what constituted cleanwater and how much water should be delegated to each family. History shows that even before industrialization andthe usage of water pipes, our ancestors were already awareof what clean water is: tasteless, colorless, and odorless. Some sources also say that our great-grandfathers would also base their determination on the temperature of the water. If it's not cool water, it's not safe water. There's an insurmountable amount of knowledge that today's technology was based on and that's what we're going to examine alongside discussing how to preserve safe and clean water.

Because people often lived as a group of families settling in an area with a water source, it was necessary for our ancestors to know how much water should be distributed throughout the community. The general rule was that everyone should have just enough for a whole family to survive natural crises like drought.

Today, a more formal note was based on our ancestors' knowledge and capabilities. The Federal Emergency Management Agency and Red Cross recommend that we should have 15 gallons of water to last us for two weeks. This means that the minimum requirement is one gallon per person per day: half is for drinking purposes and the other half is for the most basic hygiene, which certainly doesn't include a full-blown shower. If you would like to maintain your hygiene through the crisis, you might want to store up to five gallons per person per day. You might also want to consider the following when deciding how much water you should store:

- ❖ The number of people in your family
- ❖ Children, nursing mothers, and sick people, who will need more water
- ❖ The possibility of a medical emergency
- ❖ The climate in your area
- ❖ Pets or animals that you will have to care for
- ❖ The locally supplied water
- ❖ Average rainfall in your area
- ❖ Family members and/or friends that have special medical needs
- ❖ The activity you plan to do during the crisis

Generally, the rule is that you should consider all the factors that could affect your average intake of water and adjust the amount you should store accordingly.

Aside from the amount of water needed for a family, our ancestors also realized the preservation powers of silver. An interesting example was Alexander the Great who used silver runs to store water for his troops when they needed to go out on long journeys by sea. A more modern way that people used to store water was putting some silver jewelry into a storage container which effectively prevents the

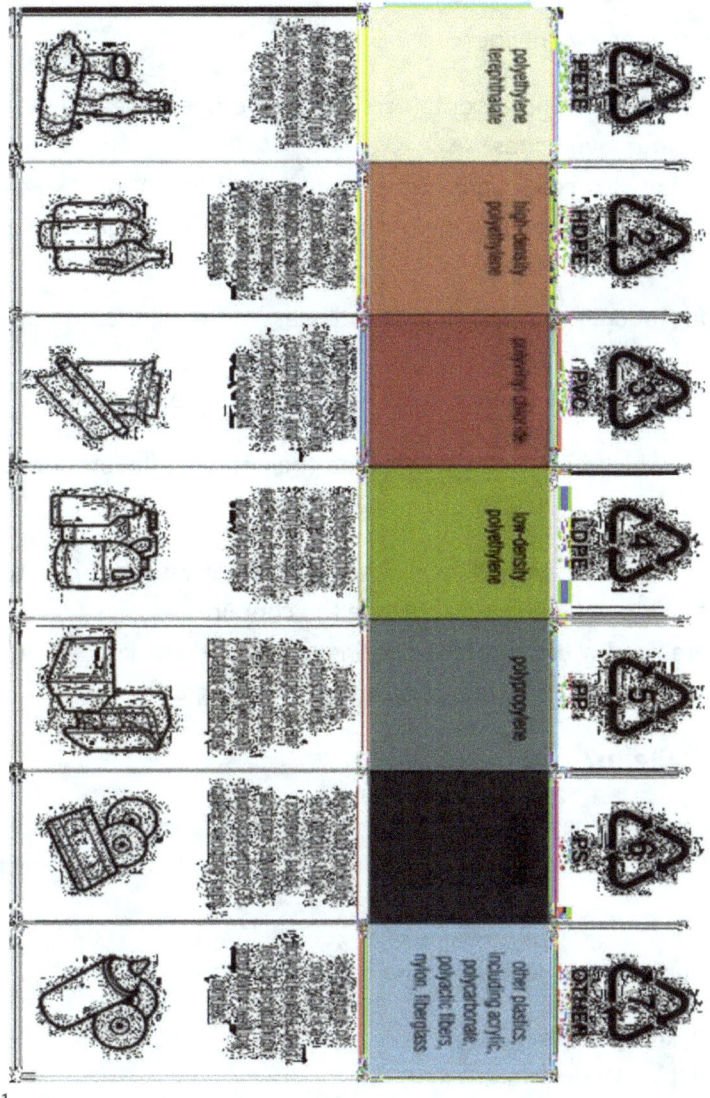

- Wash each bottle using water and dish soap.
- Sanitize each bottle and cap inside-out with a bleach solution of 1 tsp. bleach mixed in 1 quart water.
- Rinse the sanitized bottle with clean water.
- Fill each bottle with tap water.
- Add 2 drops of standard unscented household bleach (4-6% sodium hypochlorite)
- Empty and refresh your water storage onceeach year.

❖ If you'd like to be completely safe, the best containers to use are new ones.

If you're going to choose glass containers, here are some guidelines:

- ❖ Make sure that your glass container is food safe. Some containers may have been used to store chemicals, which could endanger you and your loved ones.
- ❖ Remember that glass can break easily. It can also crack under freezing temperatures. Worse, it can have tiny, invisible flaws you are unable to see that could trap contaminates in your water. Prepare proper storage.
- ❖ The best form of glassware that is safe for food and water is Borosilicate glass more popularly known as Pyrex.
- ❖ Watch out for soda-lime based glass that calls itself Pyrex as it is not heat resistant (i.e., Mason jars).

Another form of storage can be stainless steel, which was actually based on the antibacterial properties of silver. Here are the guidelines.

- ❖ Consider whether or not your water was treated with chlorine. Although stainless steel is actually more durable than the first two options, chlorine alone could corrode the container.
- ❖ It is better to look for steel drums that are lined with protective coating to lessen the risks.
- ❖ As with any container, make sure that your stainless steel containers are food grade.

How Can I Make Sure That the Water Is Clean?

The first thing to remember when disinfecting water is that you have to filter it first. Small, home filters will do. Filtering the water first will remove some of the bigger particulates and debris which will make disinfecting water easier and freer from risk.

The most popular way to disinfect water is through boiling. Here are some notes to remember:

- ❖ Water at 160 degrees for 30 minutes will kill the pathogens.
- ❖ Above 185 degrees for a few minutes will kill the pathogens in it.
- ❖ Boiling water at 212 degrees will kill pathogens as soon as it comes to a rolling boil.
- ❖ Water at sea level has a higher boiling point than water in higher altitudes.

The information above is important because in times when water is scarce, you wouldn't want to excessively boil your water until it evaporates. Furthermore, our ancestors quickly found out that boiling water was not as effective as filtration. Although it kills most of the bacteria, it isn't effective on other chemicals and turbidity. They also found out that it wasn't economically and ecologically practical as it requires extensive use of firewood and other combustibles that would soon become expensive as history progressed.

Another way to disinfect water is bleach. The history of using bleach dates back to the 1800s when a British scientist found out that cholera spread because of a contaminated water pipe. Upon his discovery, John Snow applied chlorine to water, which was as effective as the people hoped it would be. This discovery led to the first government public regulation to install municipal water filters like chlorine.

This is the process that you will have to apply if your municipality water does not add chlorine to the water supply:

- ❖ Add two drops of non-scented chlorine bleach to every two liters of water. Make sure that it is a non-additive.
- ❖ Before drinking or using the water, let it stand for 30 minutes.
- ❖ If you still smell the chlorine in the water, let it stand for another 15 minutes.

! Do not use scented bleaches, color-safe bleaches, or bleaches with added cleaners as prescribed by FEMA, as this will contaminate you water.

! Do not use pool chlorine as it is much stronger than laundry or household bleach.

Aside from household or laundry bleach, you can also use chlorine dioxide tablets and water drops. Potable Aqua tablets have been proven effective against bacteria, Giardia, Lamblia, Cryptosporidium, and viruses. AquaMira water treatment drops are EPA-registered and a single 1- ounce bottle of drops can treat 30 gallons of water.

Treating your water with iodine can also ensure clean drinking water. Simply add 12 drops of 2% tincture of iodine per gallon of water. The only important thing to remember is that family and friends that are pregnant or nursing cannot drink water treated in this process.

Distilling is another way to disinfect water. Basically, you heat up the water to the point when it becomes vapor, cool that vapor, and catch the purified water. It give you the clean water you need with the only disadvantage of the fact that it is a time-consuming process.

If you don't have that much time and money to spend on all the options above, there are ways to filter your water without making use of electricity and technology. This is based on the sand filters that our ancestors used to sanitize the water in the early 1600s and the first water filters in the 1700s that were made of wool, coal, and charcoal.

First, there were sand filters. These use the compact soil and its ability to soak in water. History records that people used to run water slowly and carefully through 3-5 feet of sand. They would boil the water after that, when they knew that the water was no longer filled with dangerous microorganisms and debris. The important thing to know about sand filters is that the top layer should be cleaned off and replaced regularly.

Another type of filter was the charcoal filters. People used to burn some wood and pick the bigger partially burned chunks out of the fire. They would then place these chunks into a bucket and pour the water to be treated into the bucket and then shake it vigorously for a few seconds before they let it stand for a few minutes. This process removes bad tastes, odors, and other pollutants that could be harmful to health.

By incorporating all the filters discussed above, here's how you can make your DIY water filter.

Materials:

- Large gravel
- Sand
- Charcoal
- Cheese cloth or coffee filter

Procedure:

- The top layer of your DIY water filter should be the large gravels to remove large objects in the water that could potentially clog up your entire water filter.
- The second layer should be sand. This layer's purpose is to catch more debris that was small enough to pass through the top layer.
- The third layer is charcoal to take out the microorganisms in the water. Crush it up to give it more surface area to catch the pathogens in the water.
- The final layer is the coffee filter or cheese cloth to catch any sediment or charcoal from going into your clean drinking water.

Where Should I Hide or Store My Stock of Water?

Our ancestors used different methods to store their water. Those that relied directly on the spring would build a small shelter over it. Because they were well-aware that water that is not cold is dangerous and would make them sick, some buried their containers underground only to be taken out when the time to use it had come. The main point that this knowledge gave us is that when storing water for the long-term, it should always be in a dark and cool place.

Here are the important notes and reminders you need to know when storing water.

- Store all survival water in a cool and dry room.
- Keep your water away from any direct or indirect sunlight.
- Mark all your containers with the date you stored them and use in rotation to ensure 1 year storage.
- Do not buy bottles of water all at once. Buy enough for each month so that you have a continuous supply for at least a year.
- Do not store your survival water anywhere near fuel products.
- Container caps should be tightly secured.
- When storing in the freezer, use plastic containers and do not fill it to the brim so that there is enough space for the water to expand due to the freezing process.
- Check for any signs of leakage regularly.

Make sure that your water doesn't become contaminated or foul-tasting. It is very important to check your containers regularly. Make sure that the seals are tight. Tap water should be changed every six months. To improve shelf-life, you can transfer the water from one clean container to another to allow some air back into it. Remember to seal it properly afterwards.

If you have silver coins, you can put one in each container.

You can also collect rainwater to use for non-drinking purposes. Although history does tell us stories of people suffering during the drought running out of their homes and opening their mouths to the heavens once the long overdue downpour came, we should remember that at the time, people were more resilient to bacteria. As technology has progressed and cleaner water had become more assured, it would be helpful to think about how resilient you might be to bacteria. Despite this, rainwater is clean enough to use for daily hygiene which can help your water supply last longer. You should also know how to get the hidden supply that's in your pipes, a knowledge shared to us again by our grandparents. FEMA recommends that you do this immediately in the event of a disaster. Here's how:

- ❖ Locate your water cutoff switch and keep your containers at the ready.
- ❖ Shut off the valve that connects your municipal water supply to your home.
- ❖ Place a clean, sterilized container under the lowest faucet in your system, and open it in the cold direction.
- ❖ Open the second faucet to push out the water.

HOW AND WHY I PREFER TO MAKE SOAP WITH MODERN INGREDIENTS

"I wonder how much it would take to buy a soap bubble, if there were only one in the world." - Mark Twain

For a long time, most people used to make items for everyday use on their own. Soap was no exception. Before industries came, people would use a variety of techniques to come up with the best smelling, long lasting soap for their needs. This skill would come in handy when surviving an incident that makes access to commercial soap impossible. It is a neat trick every survivalist and prepper should know from the word go.

History

Our ancestors didn't have the luxury of mainstream industries we've had since the industrial revolution. This means that laying a hand on lye, let alone commercially prepared soap was impossible. Processed oil, be it coconut oil or olive oil was also hard to come by. The solution that lay in the most important soap making ingredients could only be found in a natural and rather impure form of woodash and lard.

Lye is in essence a strong alkali. Hardwood ash is a rich alkali hence a sound substitute to modern day commercial lye. Passing clean water through this ash and letting it decant onto a container was all they needed to create a strong lye solution. Since distilling water was still a complicated process back then, our ancestors found their pure water in rainwater.

This process was simple and you can replicate it today very easily.

- ❖ Take a big container, for instance a bucket and puncture a couple of small holes at the bottom.
- ❖ Put a thin layer of pebbles at the very bottom of the bucket before shoveling it full of hardwood ash
- ❖ Place it over another smaller bucket that should be underneath the holes in the ash containing bucket
- ❖ Pour water into the ash bit by bit and let it seep into the collecting bucket through the tiny holes at the bottom. A quarter of the ash bucket's volume should let you collect some good concentrated lye.

Using hot water will increase the strength of the created lye.

They would then use a feather to test the strength of the lye. If the bird's feather dissolved in the lye, then it was strong enough to make soap. If it doesn't one had to boil the collected lye solution so as to evaporate a part of the water in it and make it more concentrated.

The oil, on the other hand, was made from animal fat. This could be lard or cow fat. It was heated till it melted to form clear oil before it was poured into bubbling hot ash solution while still hot. After this, the process was more or less the same to what we do with modern day ingredients.

Why Modern Ingredients

Commercial lye and processed oil increases your accuracy. It gives you pure soaps and reduces your chances of making caustic soap. This makes the process more efficient and simpler to implement. Knowing about the ash and lard approach will however keep you moving in case you don't have the commercial ingredients at your disposal.

Understanding The Process

Usually the process of making soap can be as complicated as you make it to be. I like to look at it as a simple and exciting process especially because of the fact that I get to choose all the ingredients I want to include in my soap. This is in fact the ultimate beauty of making your own soap. The ability to pick different fragrances and ingredients and watch your soap develop into something from nothing is exciting and thrilling. Coming up with the perfect soap requires you to master the art of adjustments because precision is what makes the difference between a great soap and epic failure.

However, this is not as difficult as it seems and all you need is to understand what makes the best soap through practice. You may have to repeat a procedure several times before you finally get it right. An easy way to convert the process into a manageable routine is to break down the ingredients into cups and smaller portions that you can work with. This allows you to handle the process of soap making with ease and guarantees similar results no matter how many times you have to do it. It spares you the errors of bulk soap making that can occur when you miss to make a simple portion right thus costing the entire process.

Irreplaceable Ingredients

In as much as there's a variety of soaps that people make nowadays, great soaps require the use of crystal lye or pure sodium hydroxide. You cannot replace either of these ingredients with the other because of the challenge of measurements. While there are numerous substitutes, you can never be too sure about measurements hence the possibility of making a serious mistake. Apart from the challenge of measurements, substituting your lye could also mean having soap with metallic pieces in it, which is something that you do not want. Every soap maker wants pure natural soap that is free of impurities and easy to make.

Be cautious when using lye. It eats into fabric and can easily cause holes in even the strongest materials. The same effects are also felt on the skin as it burns and irritates the skin. You need to exercise caution when using lye and wear protective covering such as gloves and eye masks to prevent the burning substance from reaching into unwanted parts of the body. Mixing the lye with water causes it to heat and fume up after thirty seconds to about one minute. The choking sensation you get is because of this process and should not be worrying as it clears in a few seconds.

Be careful not to reverse the procedure, as it is always advisable to add lye to water and not the other way round. In addition, you need to stir the mixture immediately after you have added the lye into the water. The last thing you want is an explosion caused by overheated lye that was clumped at the bottom of the mixing container. Safety being a concern for everyone, proper mixing of lye allows it to react with oils in your soap breaking it down completely. As such, you get the assurance that your finished product is 100% safe and free from caustic lye because it has undergone through the process of saponification.

Machinery and Equipment for Making Soap at Home

With every possibility of making soap exposed to you, the biggest question remains whether or not it is possible to do so without special equipment. You need to set aside items that you will use for any other purpose especially cooking. While it is possible to argue that, you will clean and rinse the items properly, take no chance. Setting aside soapmaking items is safer and more efficient. There are special materials that you could use for your needs. Enamel and steel mixing bowls are advisable to use when making soap. Stay away from plastic because some of them melt and since there is no sure way to tell which ones will it is advisable to avoid them all together. Stirring spoons could be made from silicon or styrene plastic.

For molding process, you can either buy molding items at your local store, sandwich containers or use silicone-baking pans as a substitute. The advantage of these pans is the fact that you can always peel the mold off as soon as you make it. Gather together newspapers, a quart of canning jar, stainless steel thermometer with the ability to read up to 200 degrees of temperatures, old towels and any additional additive that you may have in mind.

Possible Soap Additives

Soaps vary in color, shapes and fragrances just to mention a few things. The beauty of making your own soap is the fact that you can do practically anything you want with it. You are free to add any ingredients that please you, as well as smells that you appreciate and love. However, there are certain basic and most popular additives that you should always have in mind when making soap.

Survivalists are staunch believers in Mother Nature. Making natural soap should be a priority. The important thing with herbs is to ensure that they are properly dried before being included in the soap mixture. Some of the most common soap herbs include lavender and chamomile, although there are different other herbs that people use depending on personal preference. The goal is to ensure that you find high quality herbs if you are to make the best soaps in the market.

Essential Oils

Essential oils are gathered from different plant parts including roots, leaves, flowers, seeds and stems. Usually, fragrance oils are blended form natural essential oils or are sometimes artificially generated. It is important to know what you have. Most of the time, a recommended use of about 15 to 20 drops of essential oils in your soap making procedure is all you need to create a perfect natural soap. However, you need to be careful about your source of essential oils. Buy from a trusted vendor especially if you are keen about making natural soap.

You can color your soap as you please. Brown natural soap can be achieved by using cocoa powder or cinnamon in the mixture. Green soaps can be made from powdered chlorophyll, beetroot for orange soaps and turmeric for yellow soaps. There are many ways that you can achieve a colorful yet natural looking soap. Although some people use food colors, they are not efficient because they hardly hold color.

Apart from the obvious additives used on most soap making processes, there are other not so common items that some people use in their soap making process. You can choose to add oatmeal, aloe Vera, salt, ground coffee, cornmeal, clay, dry milk powder and other things you consider beneficial. In the end, the soap you make should be as unique as you are.

So, How do You Make Soap?

Ingredients:

- 48 oz of Olive oil
- 15.5 oz of Cold water
- 6.1 oz of 100% lye

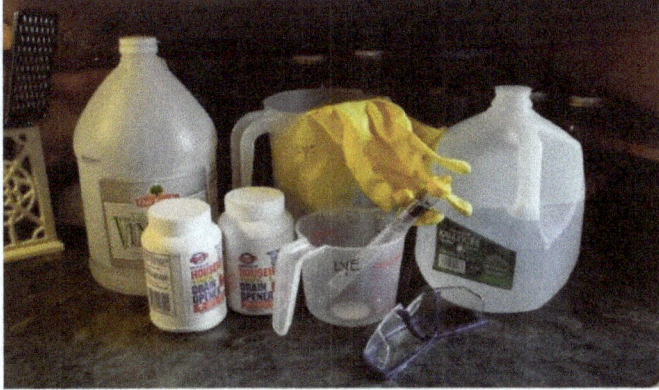

Note that the ingredients are measured in weight, not in volume. Use an electrical scale as it is more accurate. Failing to use the right weights will result in caustic or unset soap.

Equipment

- Protective gear (goggles, gas mask and gloves)
- Glass or plastic containers
- A metallic pot
- A thermometer
- Two stirring spoons/spatulas

- Small sandwich boxes to use as molds
- Plastic wraps
- A cleaver
- An accurate weighing scale

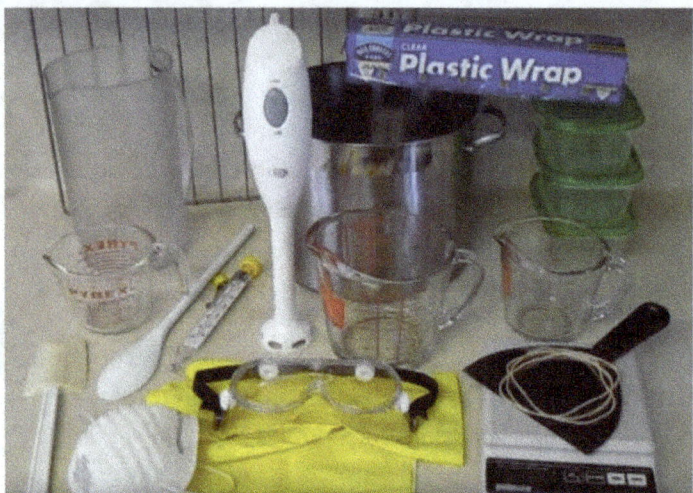

Methodology

1. **Preparing the Lye**

Lye is very caustic. You need to take some precautions when using it. Cover the work area with a newspaper – unless you don't mind corroding or dirtying it. Wear protective gear such as eye cover and gloves.

Measure water into the quartz can and stand by with your spoon ready to stir.

Measure exact amounts of lye needed and pour it into the water string with every small addition.

You should take a step back when it starts to fume and allow the gases to evaporate. Allow the water to sit as you move to the next step as the water clears. Never pour water into the lye as this could cause an explosion.

Always ensure that you are adding the lye into the water.

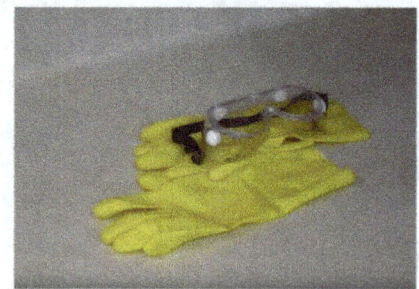

2. **Weighing the Olive Oil**

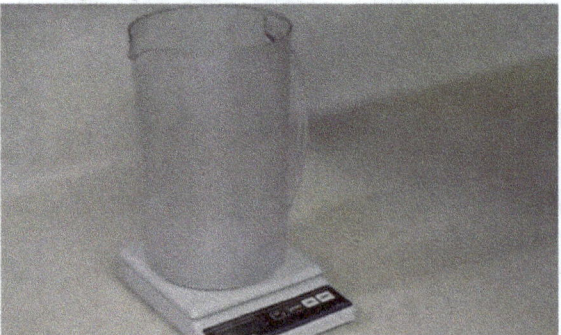

Take a clean clear jar and place it on the weighing scale. Take note of its weight as you will need this figure to get the exact olive oil weight.

Pour olive oil into the jar until it is 48oz plus the initial jar weight. This mean if the jar was 3oz, your final reading should be 51oz. Once you are sure of the reading, carefully transfer your olive oil into one of the metallic pots.

3. Heat the oil to 130F

Place the oil onto a heat source and steadily heat it to 130F. This doesn't have to be so accurate a temperature but keeping it around there ensures that you get the best results once you start mixing the ingredients.

4. Retrieve the Lye solution

The olive oil was heated to 130F to give you some ledge as you collect the other equipment and the lye solution you made before. The ideal olive oil temperature should be 110F. Give yourself a cushion that is as long as you think you need to retrieve your lye solution and a wooden spatula.

5. Mixing the lye solution and the oil

Pour a steady stream of the lye-water solution into the oil while stirring gently. The goal here is to stir until the mixture turns into a thick solution. Stirring with a stick could take you up to 30 minutes. You can use a stick blender to speed things up. Stir until the mixture is thick enough to trace shapes on its own surface. If you want scented soap, now is the time to add your aromatic essential oils.

6. Filling the Molds

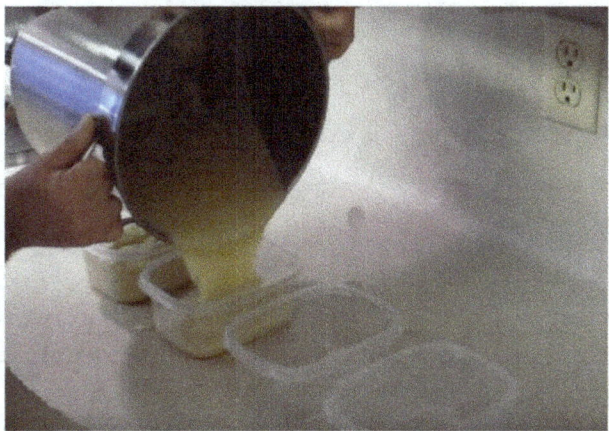

Once you have achieved a thick uniform mixture, move swiftly and pour the mixture into your mold cups. Don't fill the mold cups to the brim (you can use the plastic wrap to line the mold cups before pouring in the mix).

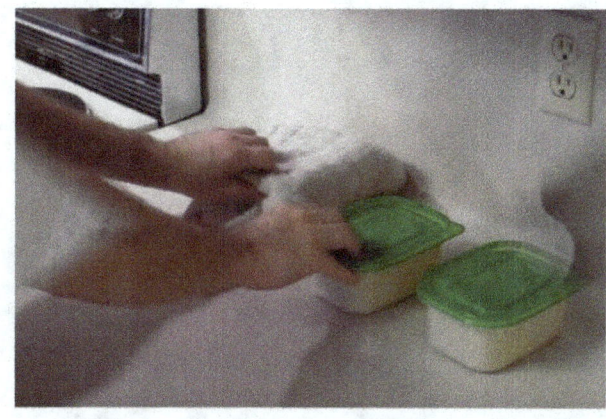

Seal the mold cups and wrap them with towels. This will let the mixture cool slowly as it sets. Give the soap a day to dry and cool off.

7. **Retrieving soap from molds**

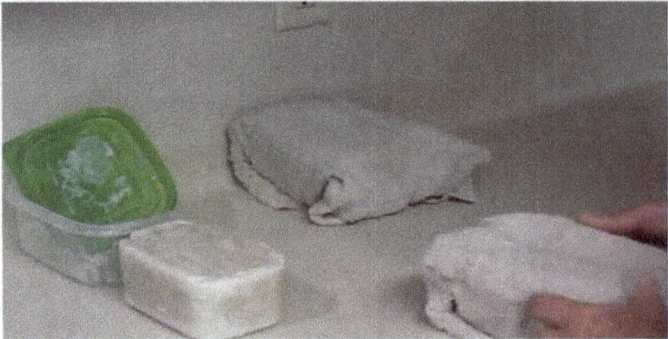

Unwrap the plastic molds and overturn them to knock out the now hardened soap. If you used a plastic wrap, this would be as easy as pulling on the wrap. If you didn't, you might need to use a butter knife to coax the soap off the mold.

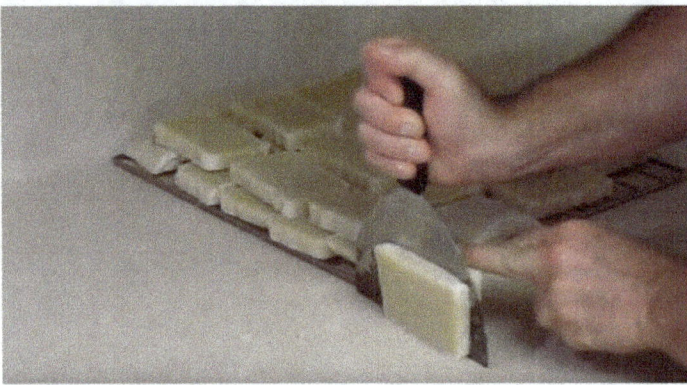

Cut the soap into a desirable shape and let it dry on a well-aerated place for a couple of weeks. Even though this step in not mandatory, it makes the soap firmer and easier to use whilst giving it that white conventional look you find on factory soap.

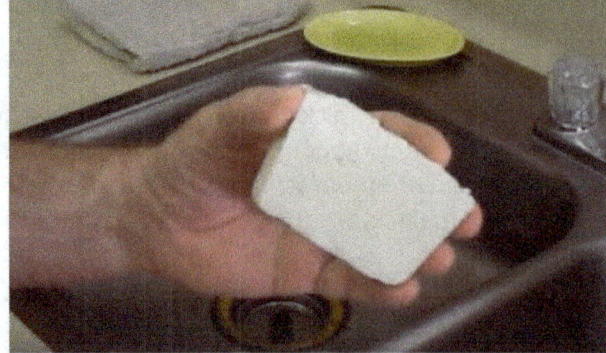

TEMPORARILY INSTALLING A WOOD-BURNING STOVE DURING EMERGENCIES

"Chop your own firewood and it will warm you twice." - Old Proverb

In the event of a grid-down situation, most survivalists are planning on heating their home with wood. That makes sense, considering the long history that man has with using wood for heating and cooking. Wood is readily available in much of the country, can be harvested with commonly available tools and produces a fair amount of heat. Although some special equipment is required to heat with wood, it is nowhere near as much as heating by other means.

For those that have a fireplace or wood-burning stove already in operation in their home, this isn't going to be all that hard to do. But adding in either one is a rather large job, especially in a two-story home. That is, adding them in the way you're supposed to is a large job. Fortunately for us, our ancestors showed us how to do this, without it being a big job.

In pioneering times, putting heat into a public building was a luxury. Many times, churches and other community buildings were built without any heat source and then the heat source was added later. This allowed them to finish the building and make it usable, without having to wait for the money needed for a large wood-burning stove.

The interesting thing is that these added-in heaters were often more efficient than the ones that were installed when the building was first built. That's mostly because of the way they dealt with the chimney pipe; in a manner that was much different than a building that was built with the stove built-in.

Why a Wood-Burning Stove

Even the earliest models of wood-burning stoves were much more efficient than a fireplace; which is what made them such a great success. The typical fireplace is set into an exterior wall of the home and only emits heat from the open front side. Some heat actually escapes through the back and sides of the fireplace and a lot of it escapes up the chimney.

This is basic physics; more specifically thermodynamics. The basic idea that heat rises. The smoke from the fire heats air, which goes up the chimney, taking the smoke with it. If this didn't happen, our homes would be filled with smoke.

The difference that the wood burning stove made, is that it radiated heat from all sides, not just from the front. That greatly increased the amount of heat that it put into a room or the amount of heat that you could receive from a log of wood.

Today's wood-burning stoves are much more efficient than those older models; mostly because of design improvements that have been done to meet more and more stringent EPA regulations. However, those regulations don't affect older, pre-existing stoves. So, if you manage to find an old wood-burning stove, keep it around for an emergency. You'll still be able to use it.

Temporarily Installing Your Wood-Burning Stove

Originally, wood-burning stoves were made of cast iron or sometimes from cast steel. Since the stove is made of metal, it gets hot. Most modern wood-burning stoves are heavy gauge steel, lined with fire brick. This doesn't stop them from getting hot though, although not as hot as an iron box without firebrick in it.

You'll need to pick a location for your stove, where it can provide heat to your room, while still being out of the way. Most people put them along a wall (in that case, it needs to be mounted at least a foot away from the wall), but they are more effective in the middle of the room. The closer to the center, the more evenly it can heat the room.

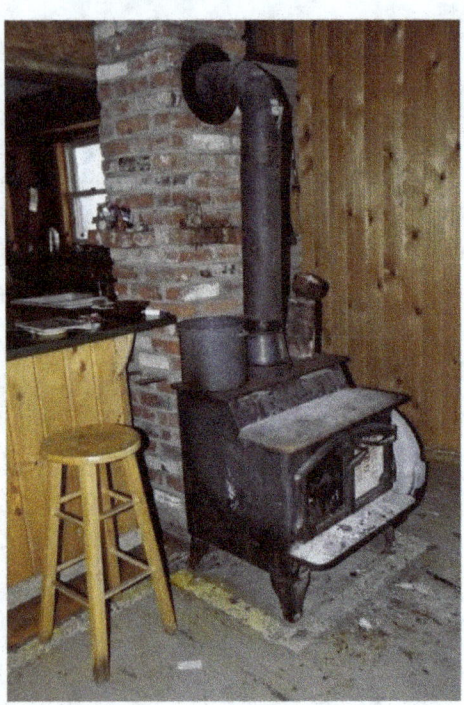

To protect your home, the stove needs to sit on a flameproof surface. This can be cement, ceramic tile, rock or gravel. For a permanent installation, you might be willing to tear up your carpet or hardwood floors for this, but for a temporary installation, you probably won't want to tear it up.

Instead, lay two layers of ceramic tile on top of your carpeting, staggering the joints so that no hot sparks can get through them to find the carpet.[52]

The tile needs to extend at least one foot around the stove on all sides and two feet in the front. Your chances of a spark are much greater in front, than they are on the sides, hence the larger area. It wouldn't hurt to go past this point, if you have space and materials available.

The stove shouldn't need to be anchored to the tile, but should be able to sit there stable on its own. Check to ensure that it doesn't rock or slide on the tile. If it does, shim it as necessary to keep it in place.

Temporarily Installing the Chimney

Installing the chimney is usually the difficult part of installing any wood-burning stove, but not so for our temporary installation. For this, we're going to take a page out of history and run the chimney the way they did in those later additions I mentioned.

The idea is to run the chimney out a window, so that you don't have to cut holes in the walls, ceiling or roof. This would probably drive any building inspector crazy, but we're doing it for an emergency situation, not a permanent modification to your home. Hopefully, there won't be any building inspectors running around then, checking people's chimneys.

There are two types of chimney pipe. In olden times, they used a single wall chimney. Today's fireplaces and wood- burning stoves use a triple wall chimney. This is done for safety, with the spaces between the walls creating a draft to ensure that the heat from the rising smoke doesn't heat up the outer layer of the chimney pipe and start a fire. But for our temporary installation, this is not what we want.

By using single-wall chimney pipe and running it across the room to the window, the chimney becomes a big radiator, radiating the heat from the smoke out into the room. That increases the overall heat you are getting from the wood- burning stove, without having to burn any more wood.

In order to do this, not only will you need single-wall chimney pipe, but you'll need a piece of aluminum flashing or sheet aluminum to replace the glass in the window. The pipe should pass through this sheet aluminum as close to the top of the window as possible and then the chimney should bend upward, with the top being above the roof of the home. Secure it in place, so that the wind cannot knock it down.

It is important that the chimney pipe angle upwards from the stove to the window, although it doesn't have to angle upwards by much. A rise of 1/4" per foot should be enough to ensure that the draw continues. Be careful to attach the sections of chimney pipe together so that they seal against each other well, especially the part that is running horizontally.

Heating with Wood

Good hardwoods will provide more heat per cord than softwoods will. Basically, the denser the wood, the more heat energy it contains. Buying hardwood firewood may be more of an investment than buying softwood firewood is, but it is actually cheaper to heat your home with the hardwood.

Most firewood providers cut the firewood to about 16 inches in length. If you cut your own, check the amount of space you have in the firebox of your wood-burning stove. Typically, there is a lot of space that is unused, because of using wood that is too short. If your firebox is 22 inches long, then you want your wood to be cut to about 20 inches. That allows you to put the maximum amount of wood in the stove, allowing it to burn longer and reducing your labor.

The wood burning stove will basically only heat the room that it is in. While you will get some residual heat in adjoining rooms, they won't be as warm as the room with the stove. This is a large part of the reason that in pioneering days, few people had multi-room homes. One large room, with the kids sleeping in the loft, was more energy efficient.

You can heat beds in the rest of your home by using a bed warmer. This copper pan is attached to a long handle and has a lid on it. Coals from the fire are scooped into the bedwarmer, which is then placed between the sheets, moving it around every few minutes. It will make any bed toasty warm in a short while.

Soapstone was also used to heat homes, as well as to provide some heat when riding in a carriage or wagon. The soapstone was heated in the fire and then placed in a wool carrier, which was placed on the floor of the carriage. Placing a lap blanket over your legs, with the soapstone underneath them provided a considerable amount of heat.

People riding in the back of the buckboard could take advantage of this heat as well, by sitting in the bed of the wagon, with their backs to the wagon seat. A blanket over their legs would help hold in their body heat, while the soapstone warmed them from behind.

MAKING TRADITIONAL AND SURVIVAL BARK BREAD

"There are people in the world so hungry, that God cannot appear to them except in the form of bread." — Mahatma Gandhi

Modern baker's yeast as we know it today did not exist until the late 1800s. Even when it became available, it was usually too expensive for most of the population, and that's why they preferred to make their own. Housewives and bakers used different types of wild yeast or massive amounts of eggs to leaven the bread. Homemade yeast could be made through various ways like using hops, potatoes, or a flour-water-sugar mixture. It could also be made from distillery barm yeast or a sourdough starter. Unlike modern day yeast, the homemade type made with sourdough starter takes a longer time to rise. It usually takes 12-18 hours during the summer and 18-24 hours during the winter. Another difference between modern-day bread and traditional bread is that the former uses more additives while the latter is as organic as it can get. Our ancestors passed on heirloom varieties of wheat to us the most common being a blend of organic spelt, einkorn, and barley. Aside from making their own bread, people from the early 1800's used to plant and harvest their own wheat.

The best time to plant winter wheat is during fall to allow for six to eight weeks of growth before the soil freezes. This also ensures proper and good root development. Planting the wheat too early makes it vulnerable to summertime insects and smothering during spring. If it is planted too late, the wheat will not overwinter well. On the other hand, spring wheat should be planted as early as the ground can be worked in spring. To grow quality wheat, here are the steps to follow:

- ❖ Make sure to do the initial plowing in the fall.
- ❖ Till and sow in the spring.
- ❖ An evenly distributed crop is achieved when seeds are divided into two parts, one part planted from east to west and the other from north to south. It can also be planted in rows.
- ❖ Cover the seeds by raking the soil over them.
- ❖ For best results, firm the bed to make good seed-soil contact.

Through constant care and attention, your wheat will grow, and you'll notice that the stalks will turn from green to yellow to brown. Once the heads are heavy with grain that pulls the top toward the earth, that's when you should harvest. To make sure that your wheat is ready for the kitchen, test out a few grains and eat them. If it's anything less than firm and crunchy, the wheat is not yet ready.

Once you've harvested your wheat, you can convert it into flour by grinding it using a hand-cranked-grinders or wheat grinders. If you don't have one of those, you can always go back to the most basic way of grinding wheat, which is to use stones or hand grinding. It may take a lot of effort and time, but the advantage is that you can control what the texture of the resulting flour will be.

How to Make Sourdough Starter (The Rising Agent People Used Before 1900)

Now that you have your flour, it's time to talk about the rising agent that most homemade bread used in the early 1800s: sourdough starter.

Materials:

- Jar or container with preferably wide-mouthed openings
- Filtered or spring water
- Flour
- Cheesecloth to cover the jar

Procedure:

- Pour ½ cup water and add ½ cup flour into your jar.
- Mix thoroughly until it feels like thick pancake batter. [53]

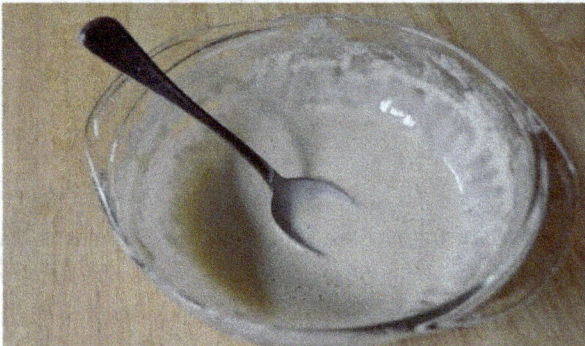

- Cover the jar with cheese cloth
- Leave the mixture on your counter for at most 24 hours.
- Feed the starter by giving it a ½ cup of flour and ½ cup of water; it needs to reach the proper

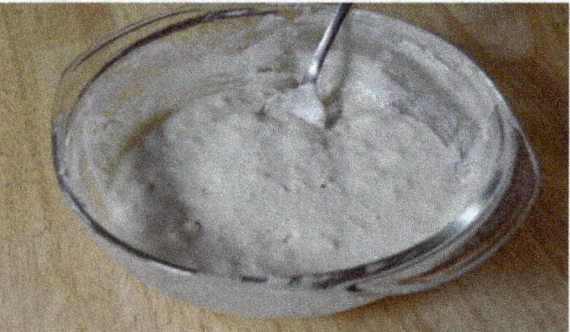

_____

consistency. By now, the start should have a few bubbles. [54]
- Stir, and cover again.
- The next day, the starter should have more bubbles and the top should look almost foam-like. Feed it again like before and repeat step six.
- Make sure to feed your starter every 24 hours. Once you notice that there is a constant rise of bubbles, it might be ready for baking.

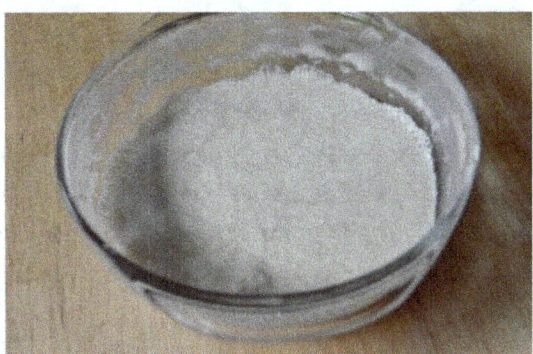

How to Make Tasty Bread Like in 1869

Now that you have both the flour and the sourdough starter as the rising agent, you can go ahead and make a completely homemade bread. The most common recipe that our great-grandmothers based their delicious bread on is "one coffee-cup flour; two coffee-cups Graham flour, one coffee cup warm water, half coffee cup yeast, a little molasses, a teaspoon of salt, half teaspoon soda dissolved in the water. Make as stiff as it can be stirred with a spoon. Let it rise over night, and bake about an hour in a moderate oven. This quantity makes one loaf." This recipe is from Mrs. Winslows' Domestic Receipt Book from 1869. A more modern adaptation of the recipe is the following:

Ingredients:
- 2 cups of flour
- 1 cup of warm water
- ½ of sourdough starter
- 2 Tbs. molasses (or whole cane sugar)
- 1 tsp. salt
- Optional: ½ tsp. baking soda

Procedure:
- Mix flour and salt in a mixing bowl.
- Add sourdough starter, molasses, and warm water.
- Stir until the dough feels wet and sticky.
- Optional: To remove the sour flavor in your loaf, add a ½ tsp. of baking soda and mix it thoroughly.
- Place the dough into a greased 9x5-inch bread pan.
- Cover with a damp dish cloth or tea towel with a dry towel over it and let it rise for 12-24 hours.
- Once it has risen, the dough should be light and fluffy. To make sure, press lightly on the dough. If it dents, it's ready.

- Bake at 350 degrees for about 40-45 minutes. If you don't have a timer, bake until the bread is golden brown.
- Tap on the bread and if it sounds hollow, it's ready for breakfast.

Making Bark Bread (Famine Bread)

Bark bread is a common form of survival food. Many would ask if tree inner-bark is really edible and the answer to that is yes, it is. It is actually a safe and nutritious wild food as long as you're using the right part of the bark from the right species of tree. The edible part of the tree bark is the cambium layer which lies right next to the tough inner wood. Edible and safe bark can be harvested from trees, the most common being Pine Trees. Slippery Elm, Black Birch, Yellow Birch, Red Spruce, Black Spruce, Balsam Fir and Tamarack barks are also some of the trees with the specific bark you're going to look for. The light inner bark of a pine tree is harvested in the spring when the bark is more easily removed from the tree trunk. Another reason why it's best to harvest in spring is because the vitamin content of the bark is highest then.

Here's how you should harvest and prepare bark.

- Positively identify the tree species
- Take only narrow vertical portions of the bark from the tree.
- Shave off the gray, outer bark and the greenish middle layer of bark to get down to the rubbery

white or cream-colored inner layer. Be careful not to shave too deeply. See picture:

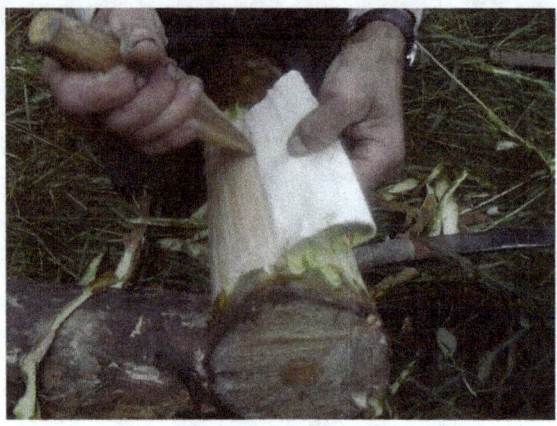
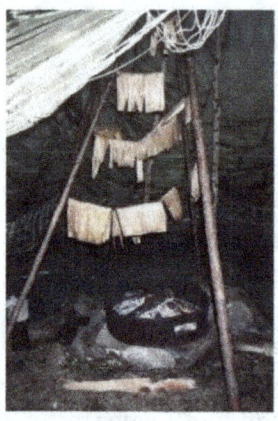

55

- Cut and peel off the whitish, rubbery inner bark.
- Dry the bark in the sun on a rack, on a flat rock, or just like in the image. It should take a day to dry the bark strips but that's dependent on the weather and the bark strip size.[56]

You can eat the bark as soon as you've harvested it. You can also fry or boil it to make some bark snacks. To make the bark into flour, you only need to dry it for a day and then pound it until it turns to powder. You can use a stone for this or a mortar and mill. The result will look more like oatmeal than wheat flour. You can add the bark flour when making your breakfast bread just like how our great-grandparents survived when they went through severe famine. Bark bread was also something that was actually part of their diet. Even during the wars in the 20th century, bark was used to add nutrition to their daily rations.

Ingredients:

- 100g or 2.5 oz. of yeast
- 1 quart of lukewarm water
- 1 quart of rye flour
- 1.5 quarts of white flour
- ½ cup of bark flour

Procedure:

- Mix all the ingredients in a bowl.
- Stir thoroughly.
- Set aside to rise for an hour.
- Knead the resulting dough from the mixture.
- Allow to rise for 45 minutes to an hour.
- Roll out into smaller rounds.
- Before baking, sprinkle with water.
- Baking time will vary depending on the size of the bread. For medium-sized bread the size of a pita bread, bake for 10 minutes at 225 degrees Celsius or 425 degrees Fahrenheit. Alternatively, you can cook the bread over hot coals as long as you turn it constantly.

HOW TO BUILD A SMOKEHOUSE AND SMOKE FISH

"Smoke Me a Kipper, I'll be Back for Breakfast" – Ace Rimmer, Red Dwarf

Fish has been part of the diet of human beings since we became human beings. Our early ancestors ate fish; the earliest form of a fishhook has been dated back to 42,000 years ago[57]. Evidence for fish eating throughout history is widespread. For example, a culture called the Etrebolle, of ancient Denmark who lived around 7300 years ago, kept kitchen 'middings' which were used to deposit their food waste. The waste included large amounts of seashells and animal bones[58]. Another example is the diet of the Mississippian culture, a Native American peoples that lived between 800-1600 AD. Archeologists have found that the Mississippians relied heavily on fish for their nutritional needs.

The reason for our love affair with all things fishy is that fish is one of the healthiest foods you can eat, containing, very little fat, but lots of protein as well as vitamins and minerals such as potassium, vitamins A and B12 and iron. The American Heart Foundation recommends you eat at least two pieces of fish per week, as the Omega-3 oils in the fish can help prevent heart disease[59]. But the trouble with fish is that it spoils really quickly and can cause food poisoning.

One way to extend the edible lifetime of fish is to smoke it. Smoking fish does a number of things to preserve it. Firstly it 'cooks' the fish and dehydrates it. Then the smoking process and chemicals in the wood smoke, such as phenolic compounds, also kill off bacteria as they preserve the meat. You end up with meat that has a much longer lifetime than it would have fresh; and it tastes pretty good too.

There are two methods of smoking fish, hot smoking and cold smoking.

Cold Smoking

So you've had a really successful fishing trip. You've got so much fish you can't possibly eat it all. So you need to preserve it.

Before you start, make sure that you smoke the fish as fresh as you can and fillet them first (don't worry too much about bones as they usually come away more easily once they are smoked).

Cold smoking is a way to add a smoky flavor to fish, whilst at the same time preserving the fish. Fish that have been cold smoked typically can last up to 7 days when stored in a cold place.

If you decide to go the cold smoke way, you must 'cure' the fish before smoking. Curing helps to control bacterial growth and draw excess water out of the fish, also helping in the preservation of the meat.

Before We Start: Woods for Flavoring Your Fish

You should always use hard wood shavings/saw dust and never soft woods. Soft woods tend to have a highly aromatic taste and can spoil the flavor of the smoked fish.

Some good woods to use and the best fish to use them with are:

- Oak – is good for smoking trout and mackerel
- Alder - is great for smoking salmon as it imbues a slight sweetness
- Beech – good for all fish
- Cedar – good for all fish
- Various fruitwoods - like plum, apple and pear are also good for smoking fish Some other woods to experiment with (depending on taste are, Mesquite, Maple and Pecan)

Cold Smoking the Fish

Cold smoking is what it says on the tin 'using cold smoke'. The whole point of cold smoking is to get a room filled with enough smoke, for enough time, to flavor the fish, and preserve it, without cooking or spoiling it. This method is more difficult than hot smoking, but the flavor is believed by many, to be worth it and cold smoked fish last considerably longer than hot smoked ones.

As a side note: Cold smoked fish, in general, do not need to be cooked before they can be eaten. However, certain of the more oily fishes, such as mackerel are best cooked after cold smoking as they can be a bit 'oily' to taste, uncooked.

There are lots of ways to build a cold smoker, this is one of those.

First Things First: Curing the Fish

When cold smoking, you really need to cure the fish first. This is a process that dehydrates the fish and prepares it for optimal smoke absorption.

- Wash the filleted fish
- Make up a cure mix of 1/3 sugar and 2/3 salt (you can adjust the amounts depending on taste)
- Place a little of the cure in a non-metallic dish and put the fillets on top of this layer

- Place the cure mix thickly on top of the fish fillets
- Weight the fillets down with something heavy (but non-metallic)
- Leave overnight
- Take the fillets out of the dish and rinse them well
- Dry the fillets by hanging inside the chimney (without smoke) for about 24 hours. You will see a kind of 'skin' form on the fish. This is called a 'pellicle' and is a thin layer of proteins, which allow the smoke to better adhere to the fish.

Making a Cold Smoker

In the first instance, you need something to act as a 'chimney'. This can be anything heat resistant.

Often people will use metal bins or even old upright freezers. The one described here was built from bricks.

The chimney acts as the smoker. It allows you to create lots of smoke, but to not get overheated.

On top of the chimney (or as an integral part as is described here) you need to build a place where the fish (or other meats) can be smoked. This is an area to hang, or a flat surface to place, the fish on.

Basic outline of a simple cold smoker:

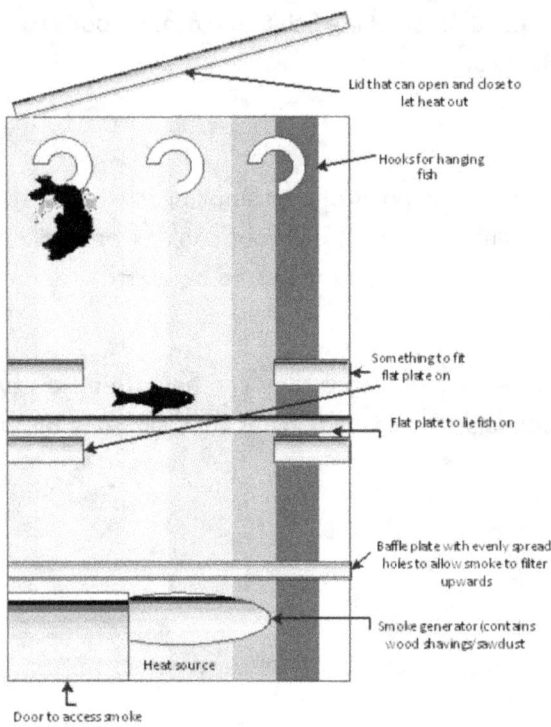

Creating the smoker

You will need:

- Bricks to create the chimney and smoking area
- Metal dish (smoke generator)

- ❖ Wood sawdust or shavings
- ❖ Heat source (small fire)
- ❖ Access door to the smoke generator
- ❖ Access door at top of chimney to control heat
- ❖ Baffle plate – with evenly spaced hole to allow smoke through (sits above the smoke generator)
- ❖ A setup to place a tray or two on for flat smoking
- ❖ Hooks for hung smoking
- ❖ Ideally a thermometer

Build your smoker as per the diagram above. In our smoker (see photo on the next page) we used heat bricks and built a short tower as per the diagram. We made sure there was an entry point to access the smoke generator and a lid at the top to let heat out.

We then placed hooks inside the smoker near the top

Under this we used metal bars to hang the flat metal plates on, for flat smoking.

A baffle plate was made from a metal sheet. Evenly placed holes were added across the baffle plate. This lets the smoke slowly filter through the chimney.

To begin smoking, place a good amount of wood shavings/sawdust into the smoke generator. You need to get this wood source smoldering to generate the heat. You can light it from above or heat it below, but getting it to smolder enough to generate smoke is the key thing. Once it is smoldering, close the access door. Keep the top lid closed too. Let the smoke build up. You should have already paced the fish in situ after curing.

You are aiming for a temperature between 70-90F. Anything above this will cook the fish and cold smoking is about preservation not cooking.

Picture of the Brick Smoker: Tim and his 'Smoke House'

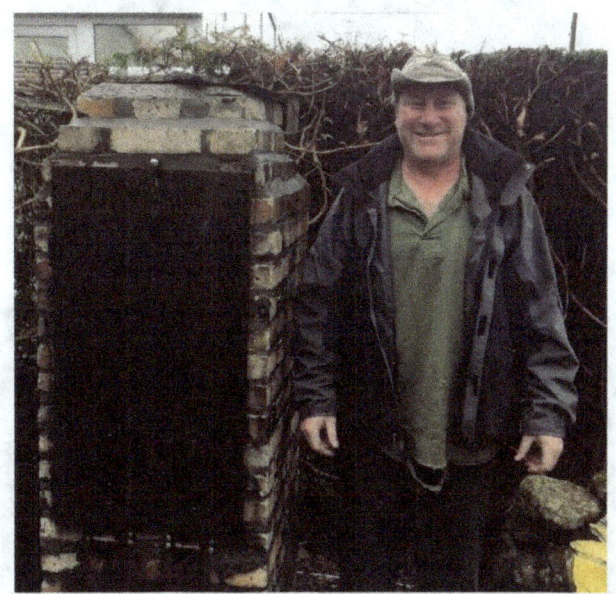

Timings

This depends on taste and on the type of fish, but typically:

- ❖ 2lbs of salmon should remain in the chimney with the smoke for 12 hours
- ❖ Mackerel or shellfish should remain in the chimney about 5/6 hours

Smoke generator (wood placed here):

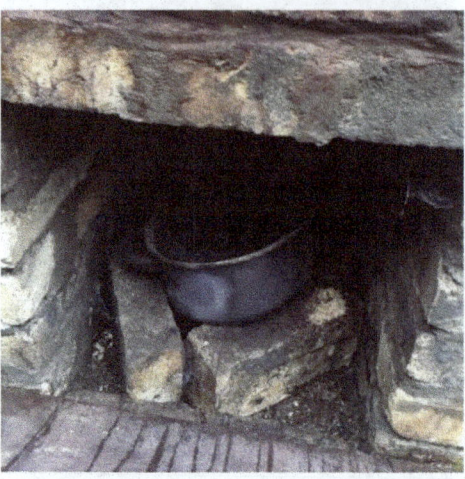

Place to hang flat plates for fish to lie on (alternative to hooks):

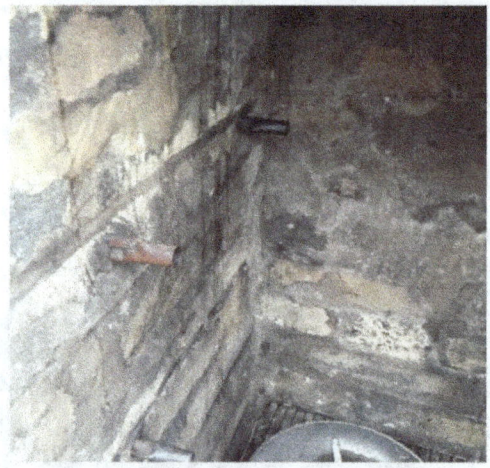

A blanket can be used to keep the smoke inside the chimney:

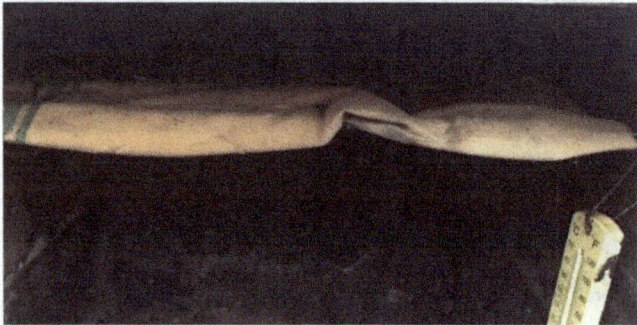

Hot Smokin'!

Hot smoking is a simpler procedure than cold smoking, but the fish doesn't last as long – perhaps a few days in a cold place.

Optional Preparation

You can smoke your fish straight from filleting, but you can also prepare the fish in a brine solution.

The brine solution is a mix of water, brown sugar and salt. The proportions of each being for around 1lb of fish:
- 4 cups of water
- ½ cup of salt
- ¼ cup brown sugar

Bring the water to the boil and add the salt. Dissolve the salt and let it cool a little before dissolving the sugar in the solution.

You can also add other ingredients for taste, such as herbs and spices.

Cool the solution down to under 40F before adding the fish.

Leave in the solution for about 2 hours before draining and drying. Do all of this in a cold area to reduce the possibility of the fish going bad. The fish will now be ready for hot smoking.

To hot smoke fish, you'll need:

- A container, preferably metal, heat resistant and with a lid (this is your smoking box)
- Some sort of trivet or mesh grill
- Wood chips or saw dust (this is your fuel) – see also 'Woods for Flavoring Your Fish'
- Heat source, such as a wood fire or hearth

Your smoking box can be anything that can withstand heat. So metal boxes like cookie tins are great, but you can use a ceramic container, like a bake ware or casserole dish, or a lidded saucepan.

Place a thick layer of sawdust on the bottom of the smoking box and suspend the trivet above this. The trivet is just a layer to place the fish on, so can be anything that is heat resistant and mess-like.

The lid needs to have some holes to let the steam out.

Place your smoking box on your heat source and leave to get up to heat before placing the fish on the trivet.

Leave the fish in for at least 20 minutes. You can leave in longer but, really timing is up to you and depends on your taste.

Notes:

- Hot smoking creates a lot of smoke, so do it outdoors or with all the windows open.
- You can throw on some herbs as the fish is smoking to add a little more flavor. Rosemary, thyme and dill are good ones to use.

Recipes Using Smoked Fish

Hot or cold smoked fish is delicious, on its own with boiled potatoes. But here are a couple of other recipes.

Smoked Trout Salad

Smoked fish is great with lots of salad leaves and herbs. This salad is one you can play with and ad various local leaves to as per taste:

Ingredients:
- Smoked trout for 4 people
- I onion
- Tomatoes (if available)
- Small bunch of dill
- Salad cress
- Horse radish if available
- Honey
- Vinegar
- Chopped walnuts or pecans

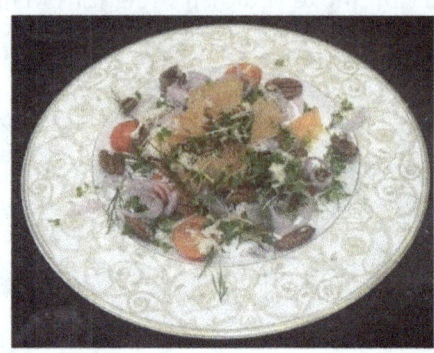

To make the salad:
- Slice the trout thinly
- Slice the onion into thin rings
- Grate the horseradish or finely slice
- Chop the dill finely
- Mix a spoonful of honey in about a ¼ cup of vinegar
- Mix the fish and chopped/grated salad items together and throw on the honey mix. Add the chopped walnuts and hey presto a delicious smoke trout salad

Smoked Salmon with Egg Ingredients:

Smoked Salmon for 4 people
- 4 eggs
- Milk, optional and if available about ¼ cup
- Small bunch of dill
- Small onions, or salad onions or chives
- Lemon (if available)
- Bread

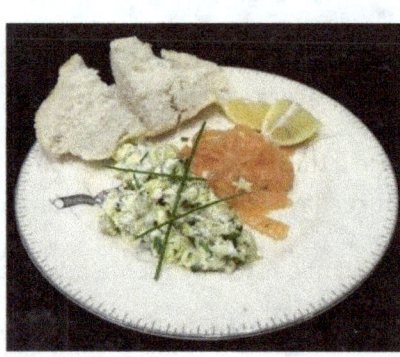

To make the meal:
- Slice up the salmon into strips
- Beat the eggs, add salt and pepper if available
- Add about 1/4 cup of water or milk (if available) to the eggs and continue to beat
- Add the chopped dill and onions or chives into the egg mix
- Add the egg mix to a hot pan. Heat the pan before adding, but don't let it get too hot. You can use oil or butter in the pan if you wish, but it's not necessary to do so. Scramble the eggs in the pan with a fork or turner until set
- Arrange the salmon strips on the plate and pour the eggs on top.
- Serve with a lemon wedge and bread

LEARNING FROM OUR ANCESTORS HOW TO TAKE CARE OF OUR HYGIENE WHEN THERE ISN'T ANYTHING TO BUY

"Take care of your body, it's the only place you have to live" – Jim Rohn

Around 10 billion pounds of soap are produced each year and in the USA about 1 billion toothpaste tubes are sent to landfill each year. We use a lot of hygiene products and for good reason. Keeping our bodies and teeth clean is a vital part of keeping our overall health good. According to the Global Soap Project 44% of deaths caused by diarrhea can be prevented through simply washing hands with soap.

So, imagine a world where suddenly our supplies of hygiene products like soap and toothpaste have dried up. Our grandparents didn't live in a world where mass consumerism reigned. They were able to create their own hygiene products from simple, readily available ingredients. It's easy to make your own products and I'll give you some recipes here that will give you the knowledge to make sure that you can keep yours and your family's health, in good condition.

Soap Making

The use of soap has a long history going back many thousands of years. The first archeological evidence for soap comes from an excavation at ancient Babylon. This soap like material was found in cylinders dating back to around 2800 B.C. (that's 4800 years ago). Soap has gone from strength to strength since then, not only being used for cleaning of humans and our garments, but also for medicinal uses too. For example soap imbued with Aloe Vera has been used to treat fungal skin infections. By the 19th century, rural Americans were making their own soap using ashes from the fire and hog fat.

Basic Recipe for Soap

Making soap is known as 'saponification'. The chemical reaction underlying the creation of soap is very basic and involves heating an oil or fat with a base (alkali) such as sodium hydroxide to produce the soap.

The more difficult of the two ingredients to obtain is the base . We mentioned earlier that 19th century Americans used ashes to create soap. These ashes were the starting material for the base, also known as 'Lye', Lye is commonlycalled sodium hydroxide and most often used in modern soaps, but if made from wood ash it is potassium hydroxideand makes a slighter softer soap.

Making Lye Water from Wood Ash

Follow this recipe to create a supply of wood ash Lye in preparation for soap making:

- ❖ Collect rain water (use rain water as it's a soft water, you should never use hard water for soap making)
- ❖ Collect wood ash from fires (the wood from broad leaved hardwoods make the best Lye, make sure itis well burned - to a white ash, if possible)
- ❖ Create a container with smallish holes in the bottom (small enough so the wood ash can't fall through)
- ❖ Take another container that the first container canfit over (this will collect the Lye water)
- ❖ Take the container with holes and cover the bottom with stones
- ❖ Fill this bucket with the wood ash to about 4 inchesfrom the top.
- ❖ Fit this bucket over the second (no holes) bucket
- ❖ Now heat up the rainwater (do not boil) and pour the water over the ashes
- ❖ Lye will collect in the bottom bucket (it's usually a brownish color)

Homemade Toothpaste

If you've ever had toothache you'll know how important it is to keep your teeth clean. The last thing you want is to have to perform 'home dentistry' on yourself or a loved one. Making toothpaste that is effective at keeping your teeth clean and healthy isn't as hard as it sounds.

If you don't have a toothbrush, use a finger with toothpaste on, or create a brush from a soft twig – chew on the twig ends to create a frayed edge and use that as your brush.

The main ingredient of any toothpaste is an abrasive substance. This is usually baking soda, but could potentially be any inert material, even clay.

Here are two basic recipes that you can use, as a starting point depending on what you have available:

Basic Baking Soda Recipe

Baking soda is a great basic ingredient for toothpaste as, being abrasive, it can be used to rub off any plaque buildup. To make this toothpaste you'll need:

- A cup of baking powder (abrasive)
- Pinch of salt (anti-bacterial)
- Water

Optionally you can also add some tastier ingredient such as mint, which you can make up yourself from mint leaves by finely chopping or grinding.

You then simply mix the baking soda and salt, adding the mint leaves if you wish. Add water to the mix until you get the right consistency for your toothpaste.

Clay Toothpaste

If you can't get hold of baking soda you can use clay. However, be careful, as it can be highly abrasive, so use carefully.

Ideally grind the clay down as fine as possible before using.

As with the basic baking soda recipe, add a pinch of salt and some mint leaves or peppermint oil if you can get it, then mix in some water to the right consistency.

To Taste

You can also add any other ingredient to create a more tasty toothpaste, this includes: coconut oil, herbs, orange or lemon peel and fennel.

Making sure you and your family are clean is the first step towards a healthy body. Even if you have the sparsest of ingredients, with a little knowledge and imagination you can produce soap and toothpaste that does as good a job as any commercial product.

HOW OUR FOREFATHERS MADE SNOW SHOES FOR SURVIVAL

"My old grandmother always used to say, summer friends will melt away like summer snows, but winter friends are friends forever."

— George R.R. Martin

Winter is the worst time to try and survive. If you think about it, back when we were primarily an agricultural society, life was built around preparing to make it through the winter. Crops were grown, harvested and preserved with the idea of making it through the winter, to the next planting season. We've even memorialized this in a way, in the creation of the holiday Thanksgiving. The Pilgrims celebrated that they were prepared for winter, and that they were going to survive.

There are many things about wintertime that make it a hard time to survive. Everything from the temperature to the lack of food is working against you. But one that we don't often think about is the difficulty of moving through the snow. Just getting around in the winter, without snowplows to clear our roads, is a bit of a challenge.

Getting around in the winter can be dangerous as well. Fighting through the snow can make you sweat, which makes you much more liable to fall victim to hypothermia. You need a way of moving through the snow, which will help keep you from having to work too hard.

Fortunately, our ancestors solved this problem for us, with the creation of snowshoes. Actually, skis were created with the same idea, but it's much easier to make and use a pair of snowshoes, than it is to make and use a pair of skis. About the only thing special you have to do to walk in snowshoes, is walk with your feet far apart.

Anatomy of a Snowshoe

Snowshoes work by spreading your weight over a bigger area so that you won't sink into the snow. This greatly reduces the amount of energy you have to expend in order to move around, while also lowering the risk of hypothermia.

While making some snow shoes ahead of time sounds like a good idea, you can also make them in an emergency situation, if you're stuck out in the woods. About the only difference is that you probably won't have as much to work with. But snow shoes are simple enough, that in a pinch, you could make a set while out in the woods that is good enough to get you home.

Snow shoes come in two basic designs; oval and teardrop. These two styles were developed at about the same time, but in different places. As far as utility is concerned, they both work about equally well. The teardrop ones are a bit easier to make and tend to be a bit longer. That's not much of an issue, unless you are trecking around in an area where there isn't much room between the trees. But then, you probably wouldn't need snowshoes there.

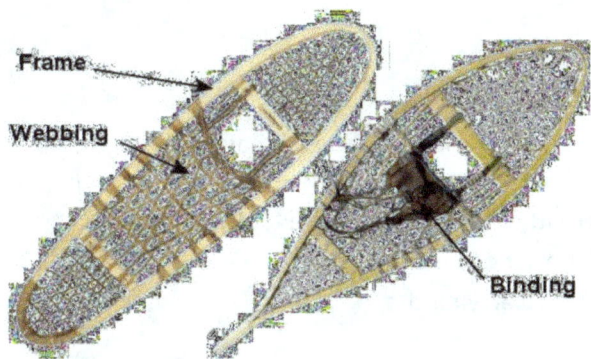

The snowshoe consists of three basic parts; the frame, the webbing and the binding. The frame defines the outer limits of the snowshoe and provides a place to attach the webbing. Crossbars on the frame help to maintain the shape of the shoe, preventing it from collapsing inward from the pressure of the webbing, as well as providing a means of transferring your weight to the shoe. When properly worn, the ball of the foot is over the front crossbar. The webbing is actually the part of the snowshoe that does the work; spreading your weight over a large area to keep you from sinking in the snow. Traditionally, snowshoe webbing was made of rawhide, but you can use just about any sort of cord, such as paracord. In a true emergency, you could tie branches from a pine tree to the frame, as the pineneedles would naturally accomplish the same thing.

Making Survival Snowshoes

To make survival snowshoes, you've got to start with the frame. This is usually made by cutting some saplings off to about eight feet, rather than using branches. You'll need to work over the saplings that you cut, making them a consistent thickness along the whole length. This step could be omitted in a true emergency, but you'll end up with lopsided snowshoes.

To bend the frames, first soak them in water for at least 12 hours and then heat them over a fire, being careful to not let them burn. If you are doing this at home, you can do a better job of bending them by clamping a coffee can in place and putting a torch inside it. The wood strips could then be bent directly over the hot coffee can. In the woods, you'll have to heat the wood and then bend it over a deadfall to shape it.

As you can see from the photo, there is actually less bending required to make the teardrop shaped snowshoes, than there is for the oval ones. Because of this, it's easier to make them consistent, a real design advantage.

With the frame bent, tie it in place. This is usually done by drilling a series of holes through the frame and then running the cordage through those holes, "sewing" the two ends together.

If you don't have a drill, a common problem out in the wild, you can heat a piece of wire, a small screwdriver or an awl and burn a hole through the wood.

Although the picture does not show it, many people will bend the toe of their snowshoe upwards about ten degrees, starting from the front crossbar. This helps you to avoid scooping up snow with your snowshoes as you walk. In order to do this, soak the snowshoe frames and heat them again, bending them over the deadfall just like you bent the frames to make the hoop.

With the outside of the frame complete, it's time to add the crossbars. These are installed with a simple mortise and tenon joint.

Cut the down the ends of the crossbar, making a shoulder in it.

Then make a hole in the frame for this to fit into. It should be fairly snug, but doesn't have to be tight. Nor does it need to be attached with any adhesive or fasteners. The pressure supplied by the webbing will hold it in place. Now that the crossbars are in place, the snowshoes are ready for webbing. If you look at the photos, you'll see that snowshoes is done in three sections. The middle it is carrying the biggest part of your weight is traditionally tied around re not using rawhide to make the webbing, you would be better off making ames, just like is done for the front and back parts of the snowshoe.

There's a particular pattern tying the webbing on a pair of snowshoes. But this is actually immaterial for a deal with this on a survival set of snowshoes is to use a simple woven pattern. It is best to weave it on the diagonal, as this will make for smaller spaces. The idea isn't so much to follow a particular means of weaving, as that really doesn't make much difference, as it is to have enough webbing to catch in the snow's surface tension and hold your weight. So, quantity is much more important than style.

You can easily use a couple hundred feet of paracord or rawhide to lace a set of snowshoes, so make sure you have plenty. You will also need a small amount for tying your snowshoes to your boots. All any snowshoe binding

consists of is a couple of straps, much like sandal straps. If you don't have leather to make the straps out of, you can use paracord.

Using Your Snowshoes

As I just mentioned, the snowshoes are tied onto the boots, usually with one strap over the toe, a second over the arch of the foot and a third around the back of the foot. However, only the toe of the boot is firmly tied down to the shoe. The rest of the binding is to keep the shoe from falling off, but the heel lifts off the shoe when you are walking.

The hardest part of getting used to walking in snowshoes is that you have to walk like you are bow-legged. If you forget that little detail, you will find that you end up putting one snowshoe overlapping the other. The first time that happened to me, I fell over in three feet of powder snow. Argh.

While you are getting used to walking in snowshoes, it can be useful to use ski poles for balance. However, once you are accustomed to them, you should be able to walk and even run, without any balance problems. The natural stride of using snowshoes is very similar to your normal walking stride, with the exception of having your feet farther apart.

HOW OUR FOREFATHERS BUILT THEIR SAWMILLS, GRAIN MILLS AND STAMPING MILLS

"It seems better to me for a child to have these skills and never use them, than not have them and one day need them" — Kristin Cashore

We tend to think of the use of machinery as something associated with the industrial age. Much of our modern tools and equipment is powered by either electric motors or gasoline engines; both inventions of the industrial age. But mankind's history of building and using machinery goes much farther back than that. Before our modern means of producing mechanical energy, manpower, animal power and even water power were in common use.

The water wheel was invented to harness the naturally occurring kinetic energy contained in flowing water. This was mankind's first "free" energy, provided by nature. Like solar power, other than the initial investment in equipment, there is virtually no cost associated with using water power.

There are three basic styles of water wheels; the horizontal, the undershot vertical and the overshot vertical. We can see an evolution of design between these three, as the most recent of the three has been the overshot vertical water wheel. However, the horizontal water wheel has been improved upon, encased and is now called an impeller. These are used extensively in hydroelectric plants around the world. So, even though it is the oldest style, it has become the only design of water wheel in common use today.

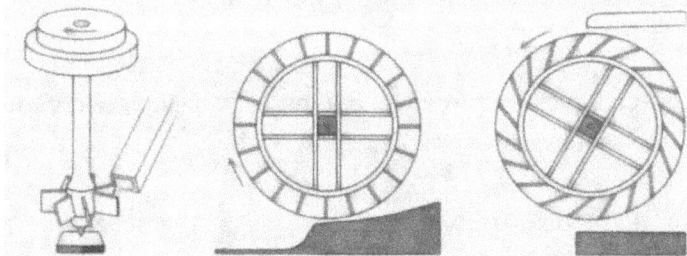

All three styles of water wheel require a channel to direct the water. With the horizontal and overshot vertical waterwheels, the channel directs the water to the vanes of the wheel. For the undershot water wheel (middle diagram) the paddles of the wheel sit in the channel.

This can cause problems for the undershot wheel, as it is affected by the level of the water. During the dry season, the water level drops, so less of the paddle sits in the water; if it is dry enough, the paddles might be totally exposed, out of the water. As this type of waterwheel works on the force of the water pushing against the blades of the wheel, the less of the blade in the water, the less power produced.

This shows the advantage of the overshot water wheel, which we want to focus on. This style of wheel is not affected by water levels, as long as there is water to flow through the channel and fill the buckets on the wheel. Clearly, this provides a great technological advantage in that the water wheel and the mill it powers can be used year-round. For this reason, the majority of the water wheels we find still in existence from the colonial and pioneering parts of U.S. history are overshot vertical waterwheels.

How the Overshot Wheel Works

I mentioned that the undershot wheel works by the force of the water pushing against the wheel's blades. The same can be said for the horizontal water wheel. But the overshot water wheel doesn't depend on the force of the water, but rather its weight.

This type of water wheel doesn't have paddles or vanes, but rather buckets. While it may look similar, it is quite different. The buckets are filled with water, as they pass under the water sluice. That makes the wheel off-balance,

causing it to turn and offer a new bucket to be filled. As the wheel continues to turn, subsequent buckets are filled, creating a great imbalance between the two sides of the wheel. This imbalance is maintained, because the buckets empty as they near the bottom of the water wheel's rotation.

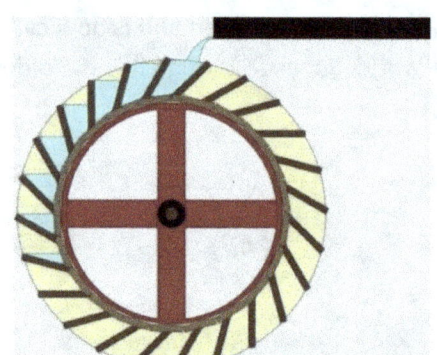

As we can see from this diagram, this leaves only about a third of the buckets with any water in them at all, and only a few that are nearly full. Water weighs 8 pounds per gallon and there are 7.48 gallons in a cubic foot of water. So, even if each of those buckets only held a cubic foot, we're talking roughly 300 pounds of water weight in the wheel at any one time.

The buckets on a typical water wheel are made by dividing two parallel wood disks into sections with boards.

The center of these disks is typically open, as in the diagram, with nothing more than a couple of beams to carry the force of the water wheel to the axle.

If the divider boards are placed at an angle, as in the drawing, rather than perpendicular to the axle, the buckets will hold more water, increasing the total weight of water available to produce force. Had I drawn the diagram above with the boards perpendicular to the axle, the water wheel would have held less than half the water in the buckets, with a correspondingly lower amount of total force available.

But that's only part of where the water wheel's force comes from. The wheel itself is a giant lever; or perhaps it is easier to think of it as a whole bunch of levers, formed into a circle. These levers are offset to the extreme, making for a very high multiplication of the force they are producing. The fulcrum of this lever is the center of the axle, with the buckets of water on one side and the other side being nothing more than the distance from the center of the axle to the far side, otherwise known as the radius of the axle.

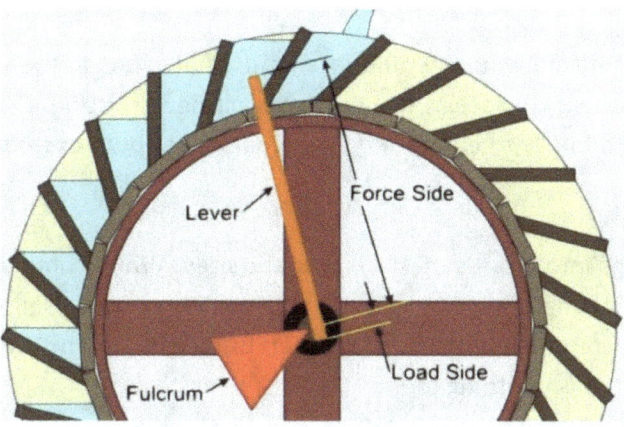

The mechanical advantage for a water wheel is easy to calculate. The formula is:

Weight of water x length (force side) ÷ distance (loadside) = Total force produced

Considering the very short distance between the center of the axle and the edge of the axle, it is clear that the force multiplication of even a fairly small water wheel is extremely high. This allows them to do a lot of work. A large water wheel, such as the 53 foot diameter Charlie Taylor water wheel outside of Idaho Springs, Colorado, can produce an enormous amount of force. This large water wheel was originally built for a stamping mill, where gold-bearing ore was broken into small particles as the first stage of smelting the gold ore.

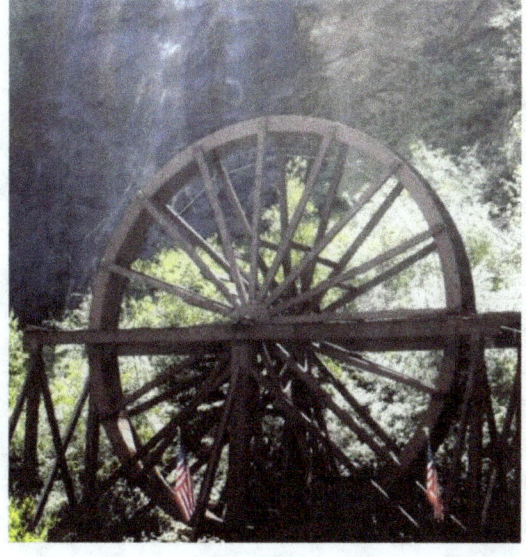

Making That Force Usable

Having all that force available is great, but it's not enough to have it at the water wheel itself. Somehow, that force has to be made useable. This meant passing the power through a gearbox, so that it could provide power in the manner needed for the mill.

Mills were the factories of pre-industrial revolution society, although not the only kinds of factories in existence. Rope walks for making rope and foundries for casting metal artifacts were common as well. But when machinery was needed, it was generally referred to as a mill. There were many types of mills, but the three you were most likely to encounter were:

❖ **Grain Mill** - Both farmers and individuals would take grain of all types to the grain mill to have it ground to flour. Hand grinding is a slow process, usually accomplished by using a stone in a stone trough. In order to grind enough for a family to eat for a day, it would take about five hours. The grain mill could do this in a manner of minutes.

❖ **Sawmill** - Sawmills cut logs into boards of all shapes and sizes. While some sawmills used circular saw blades, most used reciprocating saws, similar to a large version of today's jigsaw or scroll saw. Slow by today's standards, they were much more efficient than using a two man saw and a scaffold or splitting boards with wedges and then smoothing them.

❖ **Stamping Mill** - In mining towns, stamping mills could be heard operating round the clock. These were the heaviest duty sort of mills, tasked with breaking big rocks down to small rocks and small rocks down to pebbles.

Gears

There were a number of ways of setting up the gears for a mill, depending on the way the mill was going to be used and the time period the mill was built in. Earlier mills used wood gears, while later ones used metal gears. Metal was much more expensive, but could handle a heavier load and would last longer. Wood gears fell into three basic categories:

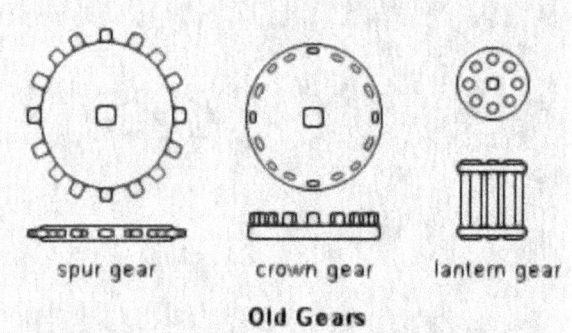
Old Gears

To protect them from the weather, the gears were pretty much always inside the mill, usually in the lower story. In the case of a grain mill, it would be necessary to change the direction of the water wheel's force 90 degrees. This was done by either attaching a spur gear to the water wheel's axle and a crown gear to the grinding stone's axle or connecting a crown gear to the water wheel's axle and a lantern gear to the grinding stone's axle.

In this diagram, the axles have been removed and the gears separated for clarity. In actual use, the teeth of the gears would mesh

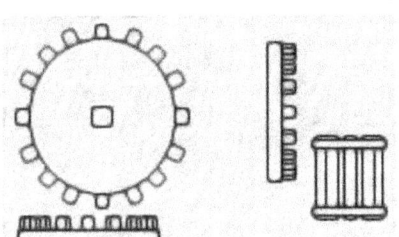

with each other. There would be a horizontal axle going through the vertical gear (spur gear on the left or crown gear on the right) and a vertical axle going through the horizontal gear (crown gear on the left and a lantern gear on the right). To allow the axles to cross, the gears would actually mesh slightly off center, as shown in the left diagram.

The vertical axle would pass through the floor of the mill, into the second story, where the milling operation would occur, regardless of the type of milling to be done.

However, gears do more than change direction, they also change speed and power. Water wheels don't operate very fast, so it is useful to speed up their operation, in order to make the milling operation go faster. So, different sized gears are used in the gear train.

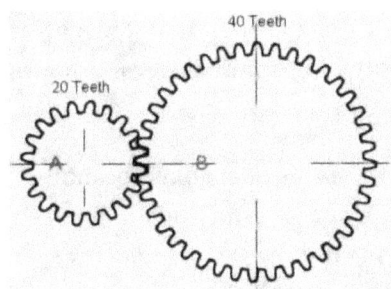

In this diagram, we see two different sized gears; gear A with 20 teeth and gear B with 40 teeth. Since the teeth of the gears must mesh, it will take gear A two revolutions for every revolution that gear B makes. If gear A is the drive gear, moving at 100 RPM (revolutions per minute), then gear B will turn at 50 RPM, half the speed.

At the same time, the amount of force that the gear is able to produce will be doubled. Put simply, the force that is transmitted through the gears is an inverse to the speed. So, because the speed is halved in this case, the force is doubled.

However, this is the opposite of what happens in most water wheels. Rather than reducing the speed, the desire is to increase it. So, the gear that is on the water wheel's axle will be much larger than the one other. It's not uncommon for the gear on the water wheel to be eight or more times the size of the driven gear. As the leverage of the water wheel produces a lot of force, the reduction of force caused by the increase in speed is considered acceptable.

At times, multiple gears are strung together, increasing the ratio of teeth between the drive gear and the driven gear. This allows much greater changes in speed than a simple two-gear gearbox. In the case of a sawmill, there is no need for the force that the water wheel produces to change direction, but there is a need for a large change in speed. So, two stages of gear reductions might be used.

In order to do this, two more gears are needed. These go on an intermediate axle, between the drive gear and the driven gear. Doing this ensures that the two gears on that axle are rotating at the same speed. If the driven gear on that axle is small and the drive gear is large, as in the diagram below, we end up with two stages of speed increase. If we assume that the gears in the diagram have the same number of teeth as the diagram above, then we are going to have a doubling of the doubling of the original speed or we're going to have the final speed be four times the original.

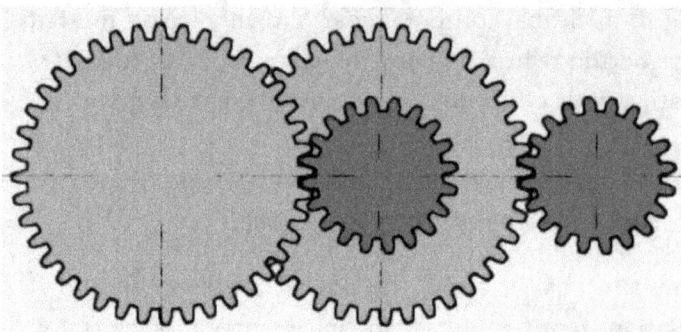

Belts

There's another mechanical device that was used in these old mills, especially in sawmills, that was the drive belt. Your car has a drive belt in it, which we refer to as a serpentine belt. It takes the power that the engine produces and uses part of that to drive the alternator, water pump, air conditioning compressor and power steering pump.

The reason belts are used is that they allow transmission of mechanical energy from one point to another, without altering that energy in any way. Assuming that the pulleys are the same size at both ends, the speed, force and direction of movement stays the same, even when transmitted over long distances.

Today's belts are made of rubber, reinforced with nylon strands. This provides a very strong, flexible belt that won't break easily. However, before the industrial revolution, they didn't have the capability of making belts like that. The technology actually came out of designing pneumatic tires, which were invented in the 1890s. Until then, belts were made out of leather straps, stitched together.

One advantage of a mill that uses belts is the ability to disconnect the saw blade from the water wheel. In this manner, the saw can be stopped, without having to stop the mill entirely. That is a nice safety feature and a fairly easy one to build in. All that is needed is an extra pulley that the belt goes around. Then, when the mill needs to be stopped, this extra pulley is moved, creating slack in the belt. The friction in the saw will naturally cause it to slow.

For Reciprocating Saws

I mentioned earlier that most sawmills used reciprocating blades, rather than circular blades. That was a simple necessity, as the amount of steel required to make a circular saw blade is much bigger. Most town blacksmiths wouldn't have the capability of working that big a piece of steel. But they could work a piece of steel big enough to make, repair, sharpen or set the teeth of a reciprocating saw blade.

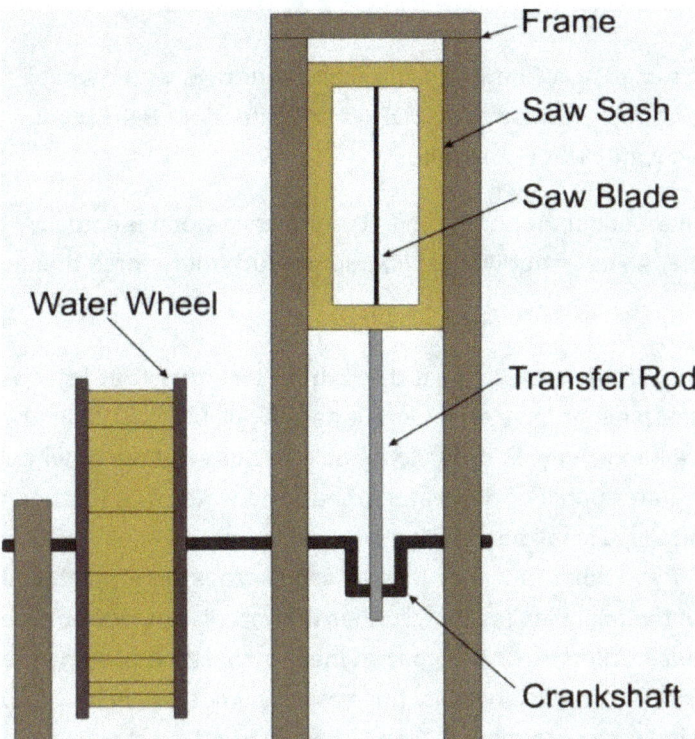

To covert the rotational power of a water wheel into the linear mechanical power needed for a reciprocating saw blade, a simple crankshaft is used. This becomes the axle for either the water wheel or for the reduction gear, depending on how the sawmill is designed.

As the water wheel turns the crankshaft, the offset portion of the crankshaft, along with the transfer rod turn that rotary motion into a linear motion. With the transfer rod connected to a saw sash, which slides in a groove in the frame, this linear motion makes it possible for the saw blade to move up and down, cutting the wood. If the sawmill produces enough force, multiple blades can be attached at the same time, allowing you to cut multiple boards.

Don't Forget Lubrication

One important item in any mill, regardless of whether it's components are all made of wood or if the gear train is made of metal, is lubrication. Lubrication does several important things for a piece of machinery, such as keeping friction down so that less force is needed to make it operate. In one case i know of, they couldn't get a grain mill reproduction to work and the only reason was there was too much friction. They hadn't lubricated it enough.

In olden times, they often used animal fat for this, rather than our modern petroleum-based lubricants. Whale oil was one of the finest lubricants available. In wood on wood application, a grease soaked layer of leather could be added in between the parts, to act as a bearing. Once metal parts became more common, brass became the preferred bearing material.

Building Your Own Water Wheel

By now, your mind is probably spinning with all sorts of ideas of how you can make your own water wheel and have a sawmill or grain mill (actually called a grist mill) for use in a TEOFWAWKI situation. Before you start, let me just add a few points on building your own water wheel and mill.

I recommend building an overshot wheel, rather than an undershot one. While the undershot one is actually easier to build, you will have times that it is not usable. An overshot wheel will also produce more force than an undershot one, making it more useful.

This means that you'll need to have your water approach the water wheel through a sluice that is at least as high as the water wheel. If you live on the side of a steep hill or have an undercut bank available, that won't be a problem. But if not, you may have to run your sluice a long way, in order to be able to build the water wheel in a position where the sluice is being provided with water uphill of the water wheel. The water that has been used by your wheel needs to go somewhere too. Typically, a small pond is dug where the water wheel is, with a canal to take the water downstream for other uses. If you don't have any direct need for that water, it should be channeled into a stream, river or pond, downhill of the mill. Plan for that, so that the water is not wasted. The easiest way to build a water wheel today is to use actual buckets, attached to the wheel, rather than forming the buckets as part of the wheel. There are several ways of accomplishing this, but basically what you want to do is to build a structure and then attach the buckets to it. Make sure that you have good bearings for the axle and that the axle is strong and stiff enough to support the weight of the water-laden wheel.

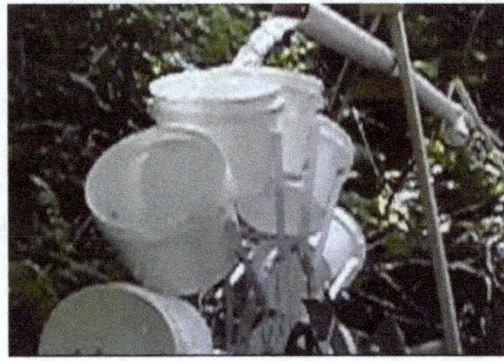 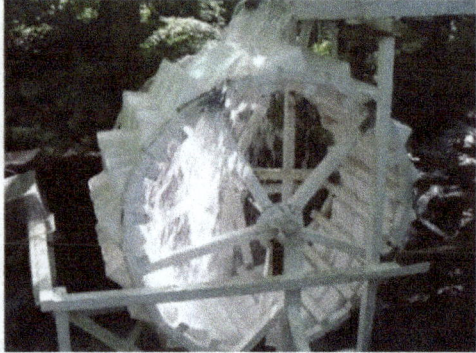

These are two modern water wheels, made by others (sorry, I didn't do it); both of which are being used to produce electrical power. The one on the left is producing 1500 watts, using about 1,000 gallons of water per hour. That may sound like a lot of water, but if you have a stream available, that's not really an issue. Whatever purpose you make your water wheel for, remember that the rest of the operation will need to be co-located with it. You really can't transfer the power that the water wheel is producing very far, except as electrical power. In a survival situation, you will want to connect any machinery to the water wheel and use it at that site.